The **Posture Doctor**

The art and science of healthy posture

If you are too damn young to feel old, this book is for you. For those who have tried numerous treatments and exercise regimes to no avail, this book is for you. If you want to be active but it hurts and for all of you who permanently slouch, I write this book for you.

Love Paula.

The
POSTURE
DOCTOR

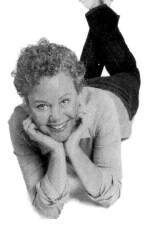

The art and science of healthy posture

Dr Paula Moore DC

ecademyPRESS
www.ecademy-press.com

The Posture Doctor
The art and science of healthy posture

First published in 2012 by
Ecademy Press
48 St Vincent Drive, St Albans, Herts, AL1 5SJ UK
info@ecademy-press.com
www.ecademy-press.com

Available online and from all good bookstores

Cover photography and portraits by Agness Lugovska
Artwork by Karen Gladwell

Printed on acid-free paper from managed forests.
This book is printed on demand, so no copies will
be remaindered or pulped.

ISBN 978-1-908746-57-3

CONTENTS

	Acknowledgements	**ix**
	Introduction	**xi**
CHAPTER 1	**Heal Your Posture**	**1**
	Step 1 (Commit To Improving Your Posture)	*1*
	Step 2 (Create A New Possibility)	*3*
CHAPTER 2	**What Is Normal Posture?**	**5**
	What Posture Type Are You?	*6*
	Sway Back	*7*
	Postural Or Slouching Kyphosis	*8*
	Flat Back	*9*
	Are You Symmetrical?	*10*
	Types Of Posture Correction	*12*
	Structural Correction	*12*
	Choosing Your Practitioner	*14*
CHAPTER 3	**How Did I Get This Way?**	**17**
	It Began When You Were Young	*17*
	Meet Edie	*18*
	Your Birth Story	*19*
	Humpty Had A Great Fall	*21*
	Meet Lizzy	*23*
	Meet Paula	*25*
	Car Accidents	*26*
	My Car Crash	*27*
	The Fatty Neck Hump	*29*
	Meet Elizabeth	*31*
Chapter 4	**It's Not Your Genes**	**33**
	Too Many Too Few	*34*
	Your Curves	*38*
	Cervical Lordosis	*39*
	Thoracic Kyphosis	*40*

		Lumbar Lordosis	41
		Scoliosis	43
		Meet Laura	43
		Betty Boops	45
CHAPTER 5	**You'll Need Help**		**49**
		Mechanist Or Vitalist	49
		Mechanism	50
		Vitalism	51
		Ask For Help	54
		Address Your Lifestyle	57
		Believe Yourself Healthy	57
		Your Body Can Change Your Thoughts	59
CHAPTER 6	**Don't Wait!**		**61**
		Relationships Suffer	61
		Meet Donald	62
		Your Kids Suffer	62
		Your Work Suffers	64
		You Suffer	65
		Chronic Fatigue Syndrome	68
		Fibromyalgia	68
		Depression	69
		Survive Or Thrive?	72
		Conditions Related To Bad Posture	74
CHAPTER 7	**Avoid Premature Ageing**		**77**
		It's Not Your Age	78
		The Arthritis Con	78
		Rheumatoid	79
		Osteo	79
		How To Stay Motivated	80
		Stop Brain Fog	82
		Healthy Tip	83

CHAPTER 8   **What About My Pain?**   **85**

Is It Too Late For Me?   *85*

Don't Wait For The Pain   *87*

What Is Pain?   *87*

Healthy Tip   *89*

Suppressing Your Pain   *90*

Your Pain Threshold   *91*

Healthy Tip   *93*

CHAPTER 9   **How Well Are You Ageing?**   **95**

The 3 Markers Of Age   *95*

How Old Are Your Bones?   *97*

Your Peak Bone Mass   *97*

Are You At Risk?   *98*

1 Your Hormones   *101*

2 How Acid Is Your Diet?   *101*

3 Exercise And Posture   *102*

Healthy Tip   *103*

CHAPTER 10 **Start To Heal Your Posture**   **105**

Step 1 (De-clutter Your Brain)   *105*

Step 2 (Think Yourself Healthy)   *107*

Brain Workout   *108*

Step 3 (Make Time)   *109*

Get Out Of Bed   *109*

Too Much Sleep   *110*

Healthy Night-time Rituals   *111*

Step 4 (Add 3 Years To Your Life)   *112*

Step 5 (Practise Saying 'No')   *113*

Meet Rose   *113*

The Helper   *115*

Helpers Beware   *115*

Step 6 (Get Moving!)   *116*

Motion Is Lotion   *116*

Sitting, The New Smoking		118
Healthy Tip		120
The 1-Minute Workout		121
CHAPTER 11	**You're Looking Fabulous!**	**123**
Make A Plan		124
Top 3 Planning Rules		125
1 Keep It Simple		126
2 Make It Convenient		129
Healthy Tip		130
3 Make It Fun		130
Healthy Tip		131
Detox Your Life		132
Emotional Detox		133
Breathing		135
Visualisation		136
Affirmations		137
Chemical Detox – You Are What You Eat		138
Other Chemical Stress		140
Your Skin		140
Move It Or Lose It!		142
Skip The Jogging		143
Healthy Tip		145
CHAPTER 12	**How Long Will It Take?**	**147**
Don't Give Up		147
Fake It 'Til You Feel It!		149
Posture Confidence		150
You're Ready-Piece Of Cake!		155
Further Resources		**157**
Bibliography		**159**
About the Author		**163**
Testimonials		**165**

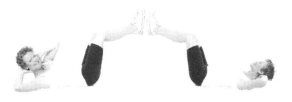

Acknowledgements

I would like to express my very great appreciation to Daniel Priestley for helping me to become a Key Person of Influence and my book coach and publisher Mindy Gibbins-Klein who provided the formula for getting the job done. I am particularly grateful to the author John Williams for writing Screw Work Let's Play.

I would also like to extend my thanks to Michael (my wonderful illustrator) who put up with my perfectionist leanings and to my book reviewers who offered their time – David Irvine, Debbie Kraft, Dem Saltmarsh, James Lovegrove, Julie Gilbert-King, Juliette Clark, Nicola Argent and Tracy Wallis and to all my wonderful clients who invited me to share their stories and pictures – Ann, Donald, Edie, Elizabeth, Elly, Lizzy, Loz, Rose and Ruth.

Finally I wish to thank my parents, Mum and Dick – my international linguists whose love has been a constant – and Nic who has been my rock, never once complaining (well maybe once) of the endless texts and emails.

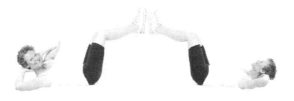

Introduction

Twenty years ago I was introduced to the idea of natural medicine after treatment from a chiropractor helped me heal the chronic headaches and back pain that I had from a condition of the spine called Scheuermann's Disease. I was amazed how quickly my symptoms resolved and decided to pursue study in the art, philosophy and science of chiropractic.

As a student, I was increasingly aware of and fascinated by all of the people I met through chiropractic who seemed to have an abundance of health and this experience was the beginning of a lifelong journey into living my own life with more vitality and joy. Over the years in private practice I had many a client that claimed to have already tried everything before meeting me and they always had one thing in common: they had bad posture.

Although some people have the mistaken idea that heathcare practioners like me are born clean-living and healthy, the truth is that most of us have achieved ideal posture as the only sustainable solution to our own health problems. I learned how to heal my own stubborn posture and I have now spent more than a decade helping people correct their posture and get lasting results where other approaches failed. I created posturevideos.com, a buzzing online platform for convenient posture correction.

Why Correct Posture?

Posture is the key to maintaining a youthful body and regaining good posture should be the goal of anyone who wants to slow the effects of ageing. This book will show you how to feel and look younger than your years. By the age of 35, many of you will be immersed in your career and the activity of your youth a distant memory. You look in the mirror and don't like what you see – someone overweight, sagging, forward head, round shoulders, stomach protruding, with various aches and pains. What happened to you?

This book does not take the place of a healthcare practitioner but may cause a total shift in how you think about your posture, health and ageing. This is not a magic cure or quick fix **how to** for the slouch potato; this is a holistic approach to understanding posture, offering a real solution to a real problem: bad posture and premature ageing. This book explains how it is that you got to be this way and even if you've never been active, your feeling of well-being that results from following the advice on these pages will more than compensate for the 'pain' of just getting on with it.

Your posture is merely a reflection of the life you have lived and the lifestyle that you keep. You will have to learn to make time to move your body regularly but I will help you to get to grips with the origin of your pain and show you how to reset your pain threshold in order to avoid the habit of medicating and masking your symptoms.

Your real age will be determined and you will be given tips to help keep your bones youthful and strong for a lifetime of exercise, vitality and good posture. It will be necessary to touch briefly on two very different health philosophies in order to make it clear that not all health professionals are on the same page.

I will challenge you to start today and I will help you to choose a structural approach to posture correction – an approach few health professionals truly understand or implement. Finally, you will get the opportunity to name your game and make a plan of action. You will start to detox your life, move your body and change your thinking until you actually believe that you can heal your posture – because you can!

CHAPTER ONE: **Heal Your Posture**

You will throw away your past relationship to health and learn to create new possibilities for your future.

CHAPTER TWO: **What Is Normal Posture?**

You will understand *normal* or ideal posture by first understanding abnormal. You will see that your posture reflects how your body has adapted to the life you are living.

CHAPTER THREE: **How Did I Get This Way?**

You will learn that the place to start looking is your childhood and even your birth. You will see clearly how the accumulation of traumas can lead to bad posture.

CHAPTER FOUR: **It's Not Your Genes**

The truth about genetics will be uncovered and you will be introduced to the spine and all its curves.

CHAPTER FIVE: **You'll Need Help**

You will decide on which side of the healthcare philosophy fence you sit and then you will learn how to believe yourself healthy.

CHAPTER SIX: **Don't Wait!**

Waiting will negatively affect the relationships with your family, your job and yourself. See how to avoid living in the decade of syndromes.

CHAPTER SEVEN: **Avoid Premature Ageing**

It's not your age, it's your lifestyle. Be aware of the arthritis con and learn how to stay motivated to avoid ageing badly.

CHAPTER EIGHT: **What About My Pain?**

Learn about the dangers of suppressing your pain and then get ready to re-set your pain threshold.

CHAPTER NINE: **How Well Are You Ageing?**

You'll discover the difference between your numerical age and your real age and then test the strength of your bones to see if you are at risk.

CHAPTER TEN: **Start To Heal Your Posture**

De-clutter your brain, get out of bed and add seven years to your life by the time you are 84!

CHAPTER ELEVEN: **You're Looking Fabulous!**

Follow these three secrets to making a plan, then begin to detox your life and get a move on!

CHAPTER TWELVE: **How Long Will It Take?**

You are going to learn how not to give up and to fake it 'til you feel it until you positively ooze posture confidence!

The website

Throughout the book I have pointed out some tools and resources on the accompanying website posturevideos. com. Go there to watch posture videos, take our free posture quiz and find further support and products for your posture and well-being.

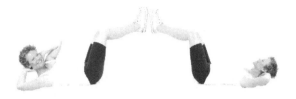

CHAPTER ONE

Heal Your Posture

'Bad posture ages you more than the lines on your face.'

Dr Rene Cailliet

Step 1 (Commit to Improving Your Posture)

Fantastic, you've done it – you've bought this book which means that you are committed to your posture and health. If you are seriously wondering how you will ever fix your posture and improve your health, just know that it starts with a commitment. Your purchase of this book proves that you are committed, so congratulations – you've taken the first step in healing your posture.

Before you dive into the meat of posture correction, I am going to help you create a *new possibility* for your posture and future health. You'll have posture that both gives and creates confidence – attractive posture that others notice. This really is possible.

With this book you can literally *transform* your posture and change your life. *Transformation* is different from change. If you simply change your posture, you might simply alter your chair position at work or sit up straight when you remember to. Change is often short-term. Transformation is about expansion (a square becomes a cube). When you transform, your feelings and behaviour patterns alter and you become more of yourself.

When you transform your posture, you throw away your past relationship to posture and to health. Do you recognise any of these?

- *I have terrible posture*
- *I want to be active but it hurts*
- *I feel old*

In order to transform your posture and health you need to begin with an acceptance of your current state of health. You must accept your current reality. Acceptance isn't resignation. Acceptance of the reality of your circumstances can provide freedom and a clean slate on which to begin a new journey.

Do you sometimes rely on painkillers to get through the day? Do you have niggly aches and pains? Do you hate your posture? Do you feel older than your years? If you are upset by your current state of posture and health, then good, that means you are committed to correcting it or you wouldn't be upset to begin with. This is the perfect place to begin.

Step 2 (Create a New Possibility)

Now you have the opportunity to create a *new possibility* for your posture and health. You can choose right now to *transform* your posture and health by inventing a *new possibility* that inspires you. You will need to write this down – get creative, this part is fun! Your *possibility* should describe an ideal state of being and may sound something like this:

*I am creating the possibility of (***you fill this part in***)*

_____

_____

_____

_____

_____

_____ *for my posture, health and life.*

Examples could include *creating the possibility* of:

- *Flexibility and joy*
- *Strength and attractiveness*
- *Youthful energy*
- *Abundant vitality*

I created *'the possibility of youthful energy and sexiness'* for myself. Now prominently display your new written *possibility*. If your words don't inspire you, you haven't chosen the right ones. Put it up near your computer, in your car, on a mirror – anywhere. Play with this and have some fun! Now before we press on and look at your posture, we will first need to understand the meaning of *normal* posture.

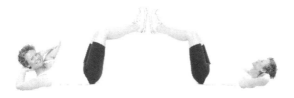

CHAPTER TWO

What is Normal Posture

To understand the meaning of 'bad' or abnormal posture we need to begin with an understanding of normal posture and ask if there really is such a thing as normal posture. Posture, from the Latin *postura*, means position. Posture may be thought of as your body position. Your posture reflects how your body has adapted to the life you are living. Your current posture is the result of the total amount of physical stress (accidents, fitness levels, posture habits), chemical stress (city or country living, food choices, household products and materials) and emotional stress from your past and present life.

No one actually has perfect posture because perfect is only an ideal. I prefer to talk about normal or *ideal* posture. By ideal posture I mean that there is an acceptable and unacceptable range of normal. You see these acceptable ranges with other population measures like blood pressure, heart rate, serum levels in the blood and body temperature. Today's sedentary lifestyle makes *ideal* posture the exception but not the rule. Most of you will have an underlying *posture type* that has developed over the years of physical, chemical and emotional stress and you are about to discover yours.

What Posture Type Are You?

Before you identify your posture type, it must be said that there are far more than the three types of *abnormal* posture that I am going to show you in this book. In the head and neck alone there are 12 possible positions (forward bend, backward bend, right bend, left bend, right turn, left turn, right shift, left shift, forward shift, backward shift, straight up, straight down). Most of you will have a combination of these positions − forward shift with backward bend, right bend with left turn etc.). There are even various combinations of three positions (e.g. left bend, right turn with forward shift).

Add together all the possible position combinations for the head and neck, add the thorax (bending, turning and shifting) pelvis and legs, and it becomes mind-boggling when you realise there are hundreds of abnormal postures you could possibly have.

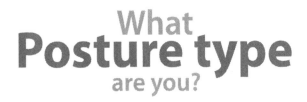

Sway Back

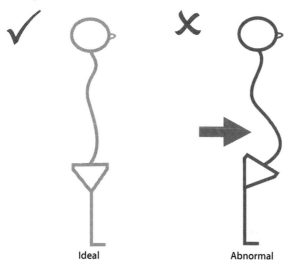

Ideal   Abnormal

- *Excessive curve in lower back (hyperlordosis)*
- *Weak stomach muscles*
- *Pregnant or been pregnant*
- *Overweight*
- *Low back pain*
- *Tight lower back muscles*
- *Tight groin/hip muscles*
- *Bendy (you might easily touch the floor with your hands)*
- *Prominent bottom*
- *Tight hamstrings*
- *A leaning back posture (your head sits behind your hips)*

Postural or 'Slouching' Kyphosis

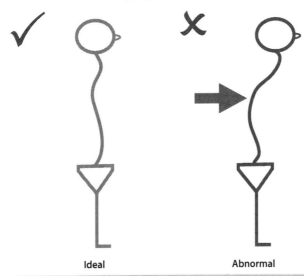

Ideal   Abnormal

- *Round and tense shoulders*
- *Fatty neck hump*
- *Slouching*
- *Forward head position (your head sits in front of your shoulders)*
- *Headaches*
- *Neck pain*
- *Stiffness*
- *Brain fog*
- *Shallow chest breathing (maybe asthma)*
- *Fatigue and low energy*
- *Sinus trouble*
- *Arm pain*
- *Pins and needles in hands*

Flat Back (also known as alordosis or without lordosis)

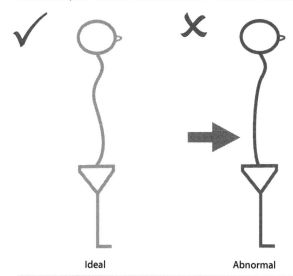

Ideal   Abnormal

- Often manual or desk-based jobs
- History of being sporty
- Flattened lower back curve
- Low back pain
- Pain when sitting for long periods
- Leg pain often described as 'sciatica'
- Pain in buttock
- Thigh pain
- Groin pain
- 'Slipped disc'
- Stiff back (especially on waking)
- Back aches when strolling
- Flat bottom

These lists are only guides. You may have signs and symptoms from only one list or a few from each list but, in general, you will have an idea of the *posture type* that is predominantly you.

Are You Symmetrical?

The position of your body (your posture) affects the position of your spine. Symmetry is as crucial to normal posture as it is to bricklaying (hence the use of a string line when laying bricks). When posture strays from the acceptable normal range, these asymmetrical loads create abnormal stresses and strains on your body tissues and this can lead to dysfunction (pain, muscle strain, arthritis and ill-health).

Good symmetry (ideal posture) allows your body tissues to respond well to stress from gravity and other forces. When you lose this symmetrical balance (abnormal posture), the stresses and strains lead to spinal degeneration (arthritis) and poor health.

Are you
Symmetrical?

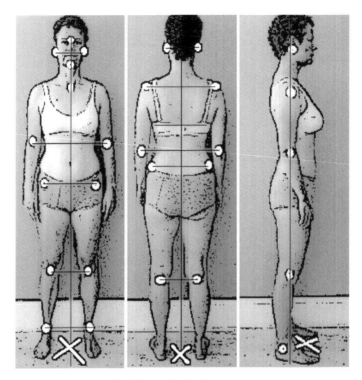

Good (not perfect) body symmetry

In the front view you see that the skull, thorax and pelvis are in alignment and the vertical line falls mid-stance between the feet. In the side view, the skull, thorax and pelvis are in vertical alignment over the ankle bone. There is a gentle curve inward at the neck (cervical lordosis), a gentle but not excessive curve outward in the thorax (thoracic kyphosis), and a curve in again in the low back (lumbar lordosis).

Types Of Posture Correction

There are two types of posture correction: *functional* and *structural*. Functional posture correction can be defined as improving muscle movement and flexibility, increasing strength and decreasing pain. This approach is often used by personal trainers, fitness class instructors and many other healthcare providers who prescribe generic posture exercises (i.e. exercises on a sheet of paper given for condition x, y or z). This approach will help many of you but more often than not you may find that your problems return as soon as you stop the exercises. Typically, you are left frustrated, wondering if you are just one of those people that nobody can help. Fear not, help is at hand.

Structural posture correction can be defined as a *programme of care* (under the supervision of a **qualified** healthcare professional) designed to change the position of the spine toward normal alignment, sometimes using traction and rehabilitation equipment. This will usually involve a detailed *posture analysis* and the measurement of any structural problems like a curvature of the spine (scoliosis) or a reversed neck curve (cervical kyphosis).

Structural Correction

Chances are good that if you have been everywhere and tried everything with little change to your symptoms and posture, then you may have only been given *functional* exercises. Functional rehabilitation exercises may improve your general range of movement (you couldn't turn your head very far and now you can), your strength, balance and flexibility. While these elements are very important, they may be missing the mark for those of you who have had little success with previous approaches. Functional exercises alone may be ignoring the underlying cause of your bad posture –the *structural* alignment and curves in your spine.

Functional (generic) exercises work really well for those of you with good body symmetry but if you give the same functional exercises to someone with asymmetry (like the woman below), strong muscles are made stronger and weak muscles weaker, perpetuating your imbalance.

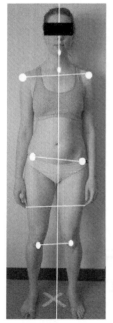 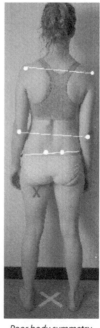 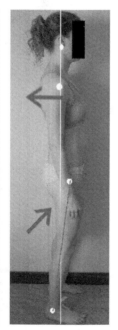

Poor body symmetry

Choosing Your Practitioner

There are very few healthcare professionals who have studied the geometry of the spine in any great detail. Most who learn about posture learn about a low shoulder, the forward head, the sway back, the weak core but few correlate these observations with what lies beneath – your **spine** and **nerve system**.

To understand the running of your car, you wouldn't make a diagnosis by studying only how the car drives or how it looks on the outside; you would look under the hood at the engine. If you want to understand a long-standing posture issue that refuses to change, you must look to the *structure* or alignment of the spine. The only way to fully understand the structure of the spine (regardless how gifted your practitioner is with touch) is to take a picture – a MRI or preferably an **x-ray** to see the bony alignment.

Not all of you will need an x-ray, especially if you have good body symmetry, but if you have poor body symmetry and have had years of ongoing trouble despite seeing numerous healthcare practitioners and trying various exercise regimes, then it is more likely you have a structural problem and may benefit from having an x-ray.

This is where the problem lies. Few healthcare practitioners have the qualifications to take or read x-rays (because it takes years of study) and often those who do believe there is no real benefit to seeing an x-ray because they already assume you have '*wear and tear*' and nothing more can be gained from viewing the x-ray. The point is there is a lot more information to be gained by x-ray examination than simply diagnosing whether or not you have *wear and tear*.

Chiropractors are trained (four years of radiology and radiography) to take and read x-rays and some, like me, have furthered their studies in order to carry out specific mathematical measurements on them. This is something only chiropractors do **regularly** and I believe it can be a very important part of understanding the underlying cause of many unresponsive musculo-skeletal problems like poor posture. I would never practise without access to x-ray equipment.

It has taken me over a decade of private practice, teaching thousands of people how to improve their posture using the same techniques I use to maintain my own posture. Much of what I know you will never need to know in order to start improving your posture and seeing results. Today I am very pleased to say that I have good posture. It isn't perfect (if there exists such a state) but it is very good. You can see my posture featured on many of our posture videos (see **Resources**).

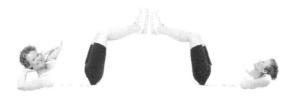

CHAPTER THREE

How Did I Get This Way?

If there is one phrase that I'd like to erase from your subconscious it's this: 'But isn't this normal for my age?' No, no and NO! I know this is what you are used to being told when you see your doctor, right before you receive pills you don't want to take. I say this because you tell me this is so.

I'm about to say something very radical: it is not *normal* for you to feel old at 30 or 40, but it's sure as heck *common*. It (your symptom) has nothing to do with the inevitability of being 30 or 40 and everything to do with your lifestyle. Many of you are spending up to 12 hours a day on your backsides. So let's be clear on this – **It's not your age, it's your lifestyle**!

It Began When You Were Young

One of the most important aspects of a posture consultation is taking a thorough life history. I really do mean thorough. I go right back to asking you about your birth if you happen to know about it. One of the reasons I spend so much time enquiring about your childhood is because your development as a child affects your posture and health as an adult. Not only is your adult lifestyle relevant to how well you age but so too is the history of your childhood.

Meet Edie

CASE STUDY

Edie is 17 years old and has suffered chronic head-aches and migraine since the age of 11. She has had brain scans, blood tests and allergy tests. She has taken her fair share of painkilling medication. On questioning her about past traumas, she seemed certain there were none – well actually one, but she figured this wasn't relevant as she was 'only five'. She described falling down hard onto her back from a jungle gym at least ten feet high. Edie's mother also recalled a fairly traumatic labour where the cord was anchored around Edie's neck.

On observation, it was immediately apparent that Edie held her head cocked to one side. It was really very obvious and, when pointed out, she and her mother were shocked that they had never noticed. We took x-rays and they confirmed what I had suspected – she had a significant reverse to the *ideal* curve in her neck (a *cervical kyphosis*). Her reversed curve is almost certainly due to her past traumas and, experience tells me, very likely the cause of her *unexplained* headaches.

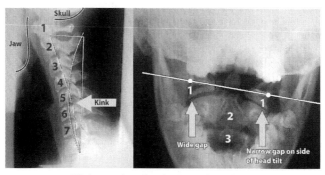

Edie's x-rays (note how her 'normal' position is bent to one side)

Neck trauma and headaches can, and often do, go hand in hand. This I know from my own personal experience of daily headaches, long before I discovered chiropractic's healing approach. You'll hear all about my story a little later on. Your history of trauma is very relevant to your current state of health. I always say to my clients that it doesn't matter if you walked away from your accident seemingly unscathed; it counts!

Your Birth Story

Your birth story is relevant to your health and your posture. Maybe you've heard stories about how you cried incessantly or how you rarely uttered a peep. Your health and behaviour as a child may give you clues as to the traumas you sustained from birth. If you were the firstborn in your family, then your birth would likely have been more challenging than the 2nd, 3rd or 4th child. These are some of the questions I'd ask you about your birth:

- *Were you firstborn?*
- *Did your mother have any accidents or back pain when pregnant with you?*
- *Did your mother give birth lying on her back in hospital? **
- *Were there any interventions? (forceps, vacuum, c-section)*
- *Were you unwell as a baby?*
- *Did you have colic?*
- *Did you have a funny-shaped head?*
- *Were you ever dropped as a baby?*
- *Did you get ear infections as a child?*
- *Did you have eczema?*
- *Did you have childhood asthma?*

* Birthing lying on your back prevents the sacrum bone from moving and opening up

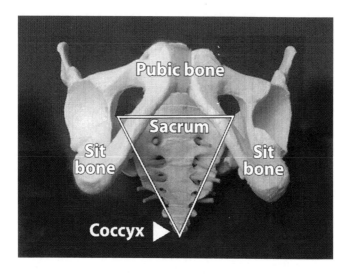

Infants have difficult births; they tumble and fall and often secretly live on junk food when at school. Parents who go to a chiropractor often leave their kids at home, even though they may have concerns about their development. I am fond of saying to 'my' parents that one chiropractic adjustment in a child is worth about ten in an adult. I really mean that. So the next time you find yourself wondering how your posture got to be so bad, look to your childhood and birth – they may provide the key to your posture troubles.

Humpty Had A Great Fall

Children fall and they fall a lot. Most falls for infants and curious toddlers occur in the home on to hard surfaces

– from furniture, chairs, changing tables, counter-tops or flights of stairs. Outdoor falls from playground equipment such as see-saws, swings and slides. Many of these falls end with head and neck injury, often unknown to the parents.

Children have a remarkable way of *bouncing* back from falls and usually walk away without all of the aches and pains we experience as adults. Some of these tumbles leave unrecognisable problems ready to rear their heads later in life. I see this every day in practice.

Do you recall falling from a height, out of a tree, off your bike or down some stairs? Have you had stitches or broken bones? I was hit on the head with a baseball bat and received eight stitches when I was 11. I'm convinced this is partly responsible for the years of chronic headaches I suffered in my 20s. Children's bodies heal quickly, often with only slight intervention. Adults take longer – often much longer. Don't forget to ask your mother about your birth if you can. Here is a little check list if you are wondering whether your child may benefit from a posture assessment:

- *Difficult birth (forceps, ventouse, c-section)*
- *You had an accident when pregnant*
- *Ongoing low back pain when pregnant*
- *Your child has/had colic*
- *Your child has/had a bad reaction to a vaccination*
- *Your child bypassed crawling*

- *Your child had a noteworthy accident (fall from a height, down stairs, in a car etc.)*
- *Your child broke a leg*
- *Your child has/had ear infections*
- *Your child was given antibiotics numerous times*
- *Your child is/was a bed-wetter*
- *Your child has/had asthma*
- *Your child has/had skin problems*
- *Your child has poor coordination*
- *Your child has learning difficulties*
- *Your child is hyperactive*

If you answered yes to at least two of these (and possibly even just one) then I would certainly consider giving your child the opportunity to have a posture assessment. Don't wait for their symptoms to begin. Isn't that what you did?

Meet Lizzy

CASE STUDY

Lizzy is ten years old. Her mother was concerned about her lack of coordination, being behind at school, holding a knife and fork, and swimming and writing difficulties. When I took her history, I took note of three significant traumas: she was glued after a see-saw came down hard on her head; she had fallen down a flight of stairs; and she had sustained a burn to her face and chest. When I examined Lizzy, she had great difficulty performing coordination tests such as walking heel to toe and balancing on one leg without significant wobbling. She stood with an obvious forward lean and she had a right *short leg*.

Lizzy has had nine sessions to date. I have addressed her nutrition, given her corrective chiropractic *adjustments,* prescribed a temporary heel lift (for her right *short leg*) in the hope of influencing symmetrical leg growth and have given her posture exercises. She has shown marked improvement in her coordination and strength, loves her treatments and takes on her home exercises enthusiastically. She is a great girl!

What traumas did you have as a child? Falls, tumbles and scrapes can cause damage to the growth plates of a bone or joint. Growth plates are cartilage plates from which new bone grows. When growing is finished the plates close and are replaced by solid bone.

'Growth plate injuries are more common in the legs and hips. The growth plate is the weakest part of the growing bone and injuries happen to active children. Most growth plate fractures get better and do not cause any lasting problems. Occasionally, the bone stops growing and ends up shorter than the other limb. For example, a fractured leg might end up shorter than the other leg.' (NIAMS –

National Institute of Arthritis and Musculo-skeletal and Skin Diseases). The resultant short limb is known as a *leg length deficiency* for which chiropractors are often ribbed about being obsessed. I have examined dozens of children over the last decade with leg length deficiencies. It is my opinion that if the short leg is noticed when the child is still growing, there is a chance to determine the cause and possibly correct it.

Meet Paula

CASE STUDY

I first went to a chiropractor in Toronto when I was 26. I initially went because of chronic headaches and also severe buttock pain having fallen on my coccyx playing ice hockey. I received chiropractic *adjustments* and my pain was quickly relieved but from time to time it seemed to return.

A few years later, at chiropractic college in England, I began getting pelvic pain. I had a set of x-rays taken of my pelvis and lower back and to my surprise I had a whopping big difference in my leg lengths – a right *leg length deficiency* of 1cm. A leg *length deficiency* is just one of the many types of *structural* problems associated with early life traumas. How many have you had?

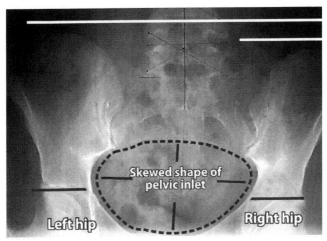

My pelvis

Car Accidents

How many times have I been taking a medical history when a patient tells me something like this: 'I did have that one accident when the car rolled but that was when I was much younger and I didn't get hurt.' Bingo! I used to ask my clients to tell me about **any** accidents they had but now I ask them to tell me about **all** the accidents they've had – including childhood, and all those from which they walked away unscathed.

After we have gone though all of the accidents, and I am always suspicious of the person who tells me they have had none, I specifically ask: "How many car accidents have you been in over 20mph?" There is a very specific reason I ask about car accidents. It was a *minor* car accident, added to the baseball bat injury in my childhood that I believe gave me years of chronic headaches in my 20s. That eventually led me to seek help from a chiropractor and thank goodness because that decision changed my life.

All road traffic accidents create the possibility of damage, whether or not you walked away. There are many factors to consider: Was the impact to the car bumper? The bumper can absorb approximately 5mph of impact. Did your head make contact with the car? Were you wearing a seat belt? How fast were you going? How fast were they going? How thick and strong are your neck muscles? How old were you? There are so very many factors to consider but I generally consider all accidents over 20mph significant. The injury is often not recognised until many years later.

My Car Crash

CASE STUDY

I was 24 years old, travelling in the passenger seat of a large gold-coloured Audi. We were merging onto the motorway when my friend suddenly slammed on the brakes, not able to merge, and we were rear-ended by the car behind. I don't recall exactly when my headaches began but I do remember a protracted period using Aspirin several days each week. Today it has been over 15 years without **any** medication.

At the age of 27, I found Dr Brian Sher (a burly hunk of a man) and his chiropractic adjustments made my headaches disappear. I was so impressed that I upped and left Canada to study chiropractic in the UK. I graduated in 2001 with a Masters in chiropractic. There was one issue, one bugbear, one total frustration throughout my chiropractic training and for many years that followed: I hated my posture. No matter what I did, I could not seem to correct my forward head posture – the posture that I believe began developing following my *minor* car accident. This *granny* posture drove me to distraction. I was ashamed to be a chiropractor with bad posture. This is me in 2006 at the opening of my own chiropractic clinic. I'm embarrassed to even show you.

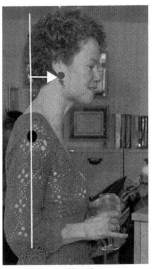

My forward head posture

I tried everything. I studied for a further two years and qualified with a fellowship in the field of posture science. I had x-rays taken of my own neck and what I saw horrified me. The x-rays confirmed what I feared: that if I didn't correct my posture, I would develop the more advanced arthritic changes my mother has due to her own long-standing forward head posture.

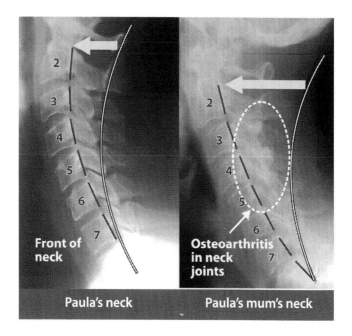

2
3
4
5
6
7
Front of neck

2
3
4
5
6
7
Osteoarthritis in neck joints

Paula's neck **Paula's mum's neck**

The Fatty Neck Hump

I get a lot of emails asking about *neck hump*. When it comes to talking about trauma (falls and car accidents), posture and how you got to be this way, it is absolutely necessary to explain the dreaded neck hump. You call it your *fatty hump, humpy, hump under neck, lump at base of neck, slight bended neck, hump at neck* and *small fatty hump*. I know you are worried about this hump. This hump is not the same as the Dowager's Hump of osteoporosis.

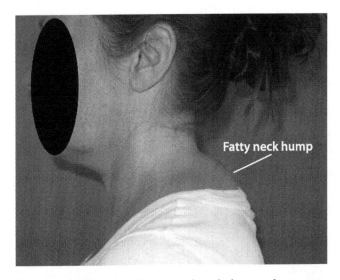

Fatty neck hump

What I describe to my clients is what I believe is the process involved in the development of the *fatty neck hump*. The fatty lump develops because of your forward head posture. Forward head posture is best described as the forward position of your head relative to your shoulders.

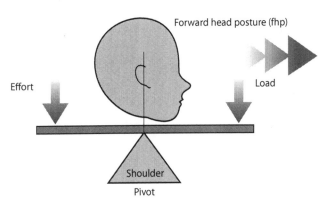

The pivot is the place where your head meets the top of your spine. Your head is the lever arm (just like a see-saw) and the neck muscles at the back of the skull and upper back provide the force (effort) to keep your ten-pound head upright against gravity (load). As your head travels forward, so does the load of gravity and muscular effort. If your ten-pound head travels forward by two inches, its weight increases to 15 pounds and at three inches forward, a massive 20 pounds! Over time, this forward head posture signals the body to lay down more fat at the base of the neck to protect the now more vulnerable portion of the spine (and underlying spinal cord) – at least this is how I explain it to my clients.

Meet Elizabeth

CASE STUDY

Elizabeth is a 67-year-old administrator and came to see me with years of 'neck tension'. She had real concerns that she was 'not standing straight', and had pain when sitting and working. The only relevant past history was that she had a severe road traffic accident at the age of 21 where she lost consciousness and had extensive body bruising. Radiographs (x-rays) were taken and the results showed what I suspected: Elizabeth had severe forward head posture causing a *cervical kyphosis* (reversed neck curve), grossly reduced disc spaces and bony fusion between vertebrae 5-7. There were no bone anomalies, making her past car accident the likely cause.

In 2006, Elizabeth was diagnosed with adult onset asthma. If you jut your chin forward as far as you can and then try to take a deep breath in you will find it very difficult. It is very hard to breathe maximally with forward head posture and it is almost certain that this forward head posture will reduce your vital lung capacity (possibly causing asthma in Elizabeth's case).

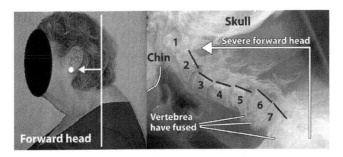

Elizabeth's fatty neck hump associated with severe forward head posture

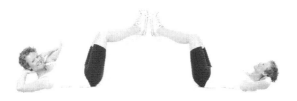

CHAPTER FOUR

It's Not Your Genes

Too many things are blamed on genetics. 'My father had a short leg' – I've heard that one plenty, but my experience has taught me that most problem posture, like *leg length deficiency*, is the result of a past trauma and only a small proportion of posture trouble is actually due to an anomaly from birth. 'When a fish is found dead out of water, do we blame its genetics or do we say it's the environment?' (Dr James Chestnut, chiropractor)

Dr Bruce Lipton is an epigeneticist and in his excellent book *Biology of Belief* he discusses and explains an individual's ability to change their genes (this is the field of epigenetics). He says that a person has the ability to change their genes by altering their physical, chemical and emotional environments. For the fish, that environment is the water.

Our genes may give us predispositions to an illness, disease or behaviour but if we alter our environment (how we think, move and eat) we can alter which genes are turned on or off. That is a gross oversimplification but enough for this book. In other words, it's not your genes!

Occasionally, it will be true – the state of your body may be blamed on your genetics. Some of you may have been born with some spinal *anomalies*. Some of these *anomalies* inevitably affect the shape of your spine and hence your posture. Most spinal anomalies are not considered cause for concern and are therefore not usually given the surgical option of correction.

Too Many Too Few

Sometimes, but not nearly as often as we think, our genetics do hold the answers. You can be born with extra vertebrae (plural of vertebra) in the spine and you can be born with too few. You can even be born with oddly shaped or fused vertebrae. The usual number of vertebrae

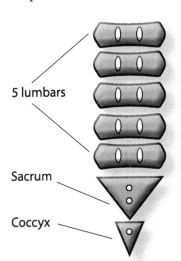

5 lumbars

Sacrum

Coccyx

in the human body is 24. We have seven vertebrae in the cervical spine (neck), 12 in the thoracic spine (mid back) and five in the lumbar spine (low back). All of the vertebrae *sit* on top of a triangular shaped bone called the sacrum.

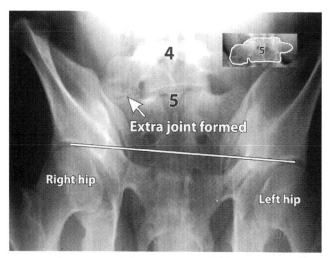

Transitional vertebra (the 5th lumbar makes an anomalous joint with the sacrum bone)

There doesn't seem to be much literature on the long-term postural effects of having too many or too few vertebrae. My experience, having had dozens of patients over the years with vertebral *anomalies*, is that these *anomalies* almost always alter posture away from *ideal*. Generally speaking, most spinal *anomalies* are considered normal variants and very rarely is surgery considered necessary.

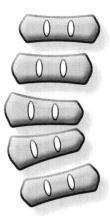

Hemivertebra (wedge shaped vertebral anomaly)

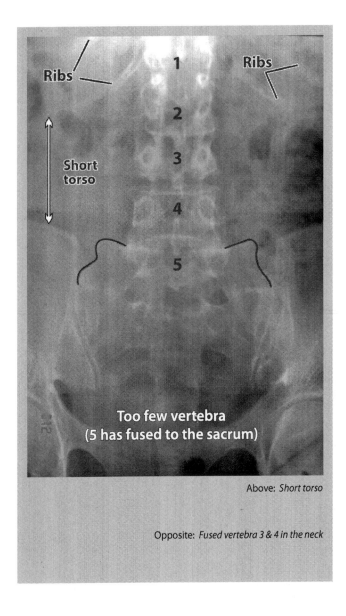

Above: *Short torso*

Opposite: *Fused vertebra 3 & 4 in the neck*

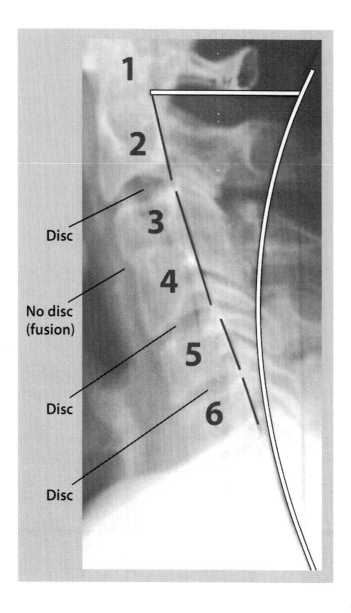

Your Curves

So now you understand that some people are born with odd numbers or odd shaped bones in the spine and even fused bones. These anomalies can be problematic if they change the shape of the *ideal spinal curves.*

The correct alignment of your spinal curves is crucial to maintaining healthy body posture. Interestingly, it is often those people who have had months and even years of treatments with various healthcare providers and still have terrible posture that later discover on x-ray that they do not have the *ideal* spinal curves.

There is much more to say on this but, for now, keep in mind that it is usually poor posture over time or past traumas that alter the curves in your spine away from *ideal.* Not all traumas will do this, but many will and certainly many more than is generally recognised within mainstream *healthcare.* Altered spinal curves change your ideal posture and decrease your overall state of health and well-being.

Recall that your spine is made of 24 movable vertebrae. Between each of these bones emerges a pair of nerves from your spinal cord. Your brain communicates with and controls the rest of your body: organs, glands, muscles and blood vessels through these spinal nerves. Sometimes the vertebrae become misaligned (often from a trauma), which *pinches* off the flow of the nerve impulse, much like stepping on a garden hose.

Think of your bony spine like the garden hose and the water running through the hose like the spinal nerves running messages to and from your brain. Trauma can change your spinal alignment and alter the ideal curves in your back, which in turn inhibits the optimum communication between brain and body and this is how your overall health is affected by your posture. So now I hope you understand why your posture is so important to good health – poor posture causes so much more than back ache.

Cervical Lordosis

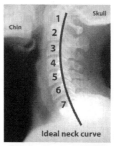

Lordosis

The cervical *lordosis* is the usual c-shaped curve found in the neck. The part of the spine found in the neck is known as the *cervical spine*. It is *normal* to be born with a lordosis in the neck. It used to be believed that it wasn't until a baby began holding its head up (at three months) that the curve went from flat to curved. Bagnall and Harris carried out a radiographic study that showed humans have a cervical lordosis (c-shaped neck curve) from just over nine weeks *in utero* and that a cervical kyphosis (reverse neck curve) is abnormal.

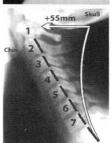

Alordosis (flat)

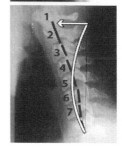

Kyphosis (kinked)

Thoracic Kyphosis

The thoracic *kyphosis* is the opposite shape to the curve found in the neck. It is a gentle outward curving visualised between your shoulder blades. The thoracic kyphosis can also be altered away from its *ideal* shape. If the thoracic curve is exaggerated we call it a *hyperkyphosis,* often mistakenly referred to as a Dowager's Hump.

The Dowager's Hump (dowager is a term from the 14th century meaning a widow with a dowry) correctly refers only to the exaggerated thoracic curve resulting from the disease osteoporosis. A person with osteoporosis has weakened bones and may develop vertebral fractures.

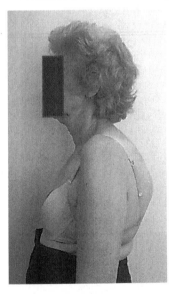

The fractured bones usually cause a wedge-shaped deformity, giving way to loss of height and a Dowager's appearance.

A hyperkyphosis may also develop through postural habit and I am seeing more and more young people every day with dreadful hyperkyphosis that I believe is happening due to the growing online social culture. I grew up climbing trees and

Dowager's hump of osteoporosis

being shouted at to 'come in'. Now we are shouting to get kids 'out' of their bedrooms; something is very wrong.

Lumbar Lordosis

You ideally have a cervical *lordosis* and also a similar *lordosis* or c-shaped curve in your low back. This curve first develops when you learn to sit upright as a baby at approximately six months. This is why your child's development milestones are so important. Holding their head up, sitting, crawling, weight-bearing and walking are crucial to good spinal development and posture. It has been my experience that children who miss these stages often have delays and coordination issues and, later, postural problems. I am quite sure that is why more and more parents are bringing their children in to see me for spinal *check-ups*.

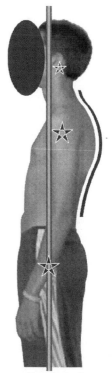

Hyperkyphosis

Just as your neck and thoracic curves can become misaligned, so too can your lumbar curve. A flattened lumbar curve is called *alordosis* and is usually a good indication of degenerative disc disease – that awful sounding term that simply means *wear and tear* of the discs. These people may have a history of a prolapsed or

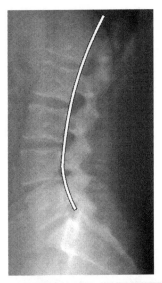

'slipped' disc and are often manual workers or people who spend many hours driving or sitting.

An increase in the lumbar curve is called a *hyperlordosis* or, more commonly, *swayback*. This posture often develops in pregnancy and/ or weight gain and generally when the core abdominal strength is lost.

Left: *Ideal lumbar lordosis*
Below: *Lumbar curves*

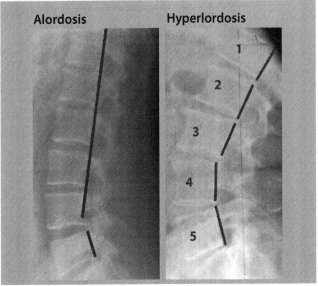

Alordosis   Hyperlordosis

1
2
3
4
5

Scoliosis

One kind of spinal curve that deserves some special attention is the spinal *scoliosis*. This is also referred to as *curvature of the spine*. Scoliosis is from the Greek *skolios*, meaning twisted or crooked. There are two types of *scoliosis* – **structural** (a fixed curve that doesn't straighten out when side-bending) and **non-structural** (a non-fixed curve that straightens with side-bending and is often due to a leg length deficiency – aka *short leg*).

The cause of a large proportion of scoliosis is unknown. Approximately 30% of scoliosis appears due to genetic defect like the ones previously discussed (particularly hemi-vertebra and rib malformations). Many more girls than boys are diagnosed with scoliosis and are usually between the ages of ten and skeletal maturity (around age 21). Interestingly, there seem to be more cases diagnosed in those who have high arches. Other causes of scoliosis include nerve or muscle disease, infection, radiation, trauma, tumour and arthritic joint disease.

Meet Laura

CASE STUDY

Laura, a slim 21-year-old student, came to me with a five-year history of low back pain. She was worried because she had been told she had a scoliosis at the age of 19. She was experiencing a 'deep constant ache' that was getting worse. Previous treatments had been unsuccessful. She recalled only one significant trauma, aged nine, when she fell hard on to her back from a radiator. On observation, it was very clear that she had a rather large scoliosis. I sent her for an immediate x-ray and it showed a large double scoliosis with a measured left *leg length deficiency* of 9mm and a corresponding drop in her pelvis to the short leg side.

As Laura's spinal curvature bends toward the side of her short leg (the left), it was appropriate for me to use a heel lift. The heel lift was used to give her 5mm of height on the short left side. This lift helps to *prop* the dropped pelvis, thereby relieving some of her constant muscle strain. Using the heel lift, along with regular chiropractic adjustments through the stiff joints of her scoliosis, helps to keep Laura free of pain.

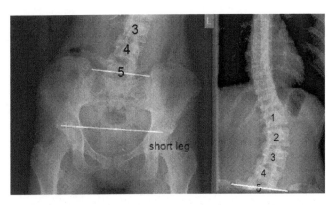

Laura's x-rays (she is facing you)

I have been using heels lifts in practice for over a decade and first began by using myself as the guinea pig. You will recall I have a right *leg length deficiency* of 1cm (10mm).

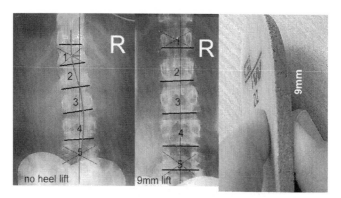

My spine straightens when using the heel lift

Betty Boops

Now depending on how some of you look at it, you were either blessed or cursed with a large chest size and yes, you can blame this one on your genes. You may have memories of unwanted attention and this often created a shrinking, wary introvert. I didn't have that problem. I have memories of running around my back garden topless (aged 14 no less) and then crying to my father when I got teased. I was a late developer.

Some of you learned to hide your feminine curves by slouching. This learned behaviour for some of you was never addressed and now you have the adult posture of a bashful, hesitant, unconfident woman trying to make it in a world where posture speaks volumes about who you are. Soon I will teach you how to change that.

If your body developed early you may have experienced being bullied at school. Bullying seems to be the buzz word of the 21st century but of course it has been around for donkey's years. Bullying can be name-calling, physical, social, homophobic, cyber, racist or sexist. The victim often responds to bullying by becoming invisible. In the animal community we would witness cowering. Victims of bullying learn to cower with their posture. They slouch and hide themselves, hoping not to be noticed. This pattern of behaviour over time can become a permanent posture. You try to *sit up straight* but it hurts. You eventually slouch again finding this posture less painful and less tiring. You email me with these descriptive words of concern: *slumping forward, slouching back, Dowager's, hunch back, slouchy, hunched over* and *hunching.*

So when you next stop and ponder 'How did I get this way?' you should now understand that it began when you were young – at your birth, through the many falls and tumbles of childhood, the traumas you have sustained as an adult and the slouching postures that accompany your insecurities and lifestyle. You recognise that those traumas and postures have affected your body shape and spinal curves over time. For a minority of you, your genetics may have played a role in changing the curves in your spine, but largely you have the ability to change your genetics and health by altering your physical, chemical and emotional environments. So even if it didn't all start out just right, it's not all doom and gloom because good body posture and health can be practised and learned.

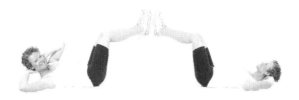

CHAPTER FIVE

You'll Need Help

You'd like to get healthy but who is out there to help you? If you decide to ask somebody for help, and some of you may choose to go it alone, you'll need to decide what side of the healthcare philosophy fence you sit.

Mechanist Or Vitalist?

When it comes to the philosophy of health, we can broadly define two schools of thought: **mechanism** and **vitalism**. 'Vitalism respects the structure and function of living things while at the same time recognising that there is an "innate intelligence" that designed and keeps the systems working as they should.' (Dr Sarah Farrant, author of *The Vital Truth*) Mechanism looks at the function of living things as the sum of their parts; the parts are seen in isolation and there is no sense of *intelligence* or whole.

The mechanistic philosophy (sometimes known as reductionist or allopathic) looks at the body as a machine of sorts. If the machine is broken, we can repair the part (or remove the part) and often without consideration of the other parts. The part is considered faulty and therefore the source of the problem. This *theory* seems valid but starts to falter when we compare the human body to a machine. The mechanistic philosophy maintains that the body needs outside intervention. In other words, we are powerless and do not have an innate ability to heal ourselves.

The mechanists believe in medicating. Medication is used to *fix* a problem – usually to get rid of a sign like high blood pressure or to remove a symptom (ache or pain). This reliance on *fixing* places more value on the outside fixer and less on our own body's ability to heal – a body that actually made itself!

Mechanism

Moving away from relying so heavily on medication would certainly be a very holistic way to approach health and yet there is one mainstream health philosophy that continues to use medication as the first port of call.

The Journal of the American Medical Association (JAMA) published an extensive study that revealed '106,000 people die annually in American hospitals from medication side effects. Medication reactions are the fourth leading cause of death in the United States, dwarfing the number of deaths caused by automobile accidents, AIDS, alcohol and illicit drug abuses, infectious diseases, diabetes, and murder.' (Dr Jay S Cohen, author of *Overdose*)

Now I'm not advocating everyone stops taking their medication – so don't! What I am suggesting is that we need a new way of looking at the health of our bodies. Perhaps we need a total shift in thinking about health and how much say we might actually have in how things turn out for us. More knowledge means more informed choice. I do believe that we all have a choice when it comes to what we do to and with our bodies.

The mechanistic viewpoint (the *fix*) was highly regarded in the early 1930s until Albert Einstein discovered that matter was made mostly of *empty* space or energy. This energy was critical for keeping the matter together. It was about this time that the vitalistic philosophy was born.

Vitalism

Today, people are making more choices about their own health care. No longer will we accept a system of healthcare where we are talked down to. We want to be involved and understand our health and well-being. Vitalists understand that there is something, some *life force,* an energy as Einstein discovered, that organises the human body and keeps us alive.

Vitalism, however, isn't some New Age fluffy science. Vitalism has been around since Hippocrates (the father of western medicine). Hippocrates strongly believed in vitalism. He believed that the body functioned as one whole organism (not a series of parts) and must be treated as a whole in health and in disease. Hippocrates proved that disease and illness and signs and symptoms were normal body processes. He believed that *dis-ease* resulted from an imbalance within the body and that the role of the physician was to restore health by restoring balance to the whole body.

The World Health Organisation defines health as, 'a state of complete physical, mental, and social well-being and not merely the absence of disease or infirmity'. Somewhere along the way we have lost this vitalistic philosophy. Clearly, your well-being is **not** merely down to the absence of aches and pains. It is possible to have no pain and still be unhealthy just as it is very possible to have pain and be entirely healthy.

> *A true vitalistic philosophy*
> *addresses the whole person.*

Once you understand this vitalistic philosophy of health, you may desire support from a healthcare discipline that is intrinsically vitalistic. For me that discipline is chiropractic but I by no means feel that everyone requires the same *medicine*. A true vitalistic philosophy addresses the whole person. A vitalistic healthcare provider will look at your physical, chemical and emotional environment and approach disease and illness by addressing all three.

Physical	Chemical	Emotional
Accidents and trauma	Nutrition	Relationships
Posture	Hydration	Ability to slow down
Exercise	Toxins (cosmetics, detergents)	Self expression
Treatments	Environment (allergens, emissions)	Diaphragm breathing
Therapy		

Mechanism	Vitalism
No innate or inborn body intelligence	Life is sustained by a vital force (Einstein's energy)
Outside-in approach to health (surgery, drugs, food, exercise)	Health from the inside coordinated by a healthy nerve system
You're a passive participant and fear signs and symptoms	You are an active participant and trust your body to heal
Your body is just the sum of its parts (like a machine)	You are greater than your parts (an inborn energy exists)
Disease is bad and needs eradication	Disease is a necessary part of health

Ask For Help

Some of you may choose to go it alone and others of you may find you go farther with support. As much as my work involves being with others in a *team*, I'm not a natural team player. I suppose I'm just too darn controlling to relinquish that authority and put the fate of my success in the hands of another. Don't be this stubborn!

If I reflect on the times when I have been most successful in my life it is because I have had support. The writing of this book is happening because I have a book coach. For my own healthcare I also have support. I've always been fairly motivated to exercise because I love how my body and mind feel with regular movement. I have regular support to assist my body in maintaining a state of optimum health. I have a bi-monthly adjustment from my chiropractor and a monthly deep tissue massage. My entire family receive regular chiropractic check-ups.

There are numerous approaches out there for natural health care. Choose one that resonates with you. If you don't enjoy it you won't benefit from it fully and you will likely stop going. People ask me questions like, "Will I need to go forever?". The simple answer is 'no!'

If your teeth feel good and seem healthy, do you still want to get them checked and maintained? The vast majority of you probably get your teeth checked regularly, so why wouldn't you like to give your body the same attention? When you stop treatment is **always** up to you. I have received chiropractic care for over 20 years and had regular massage for almost ten years and I have no plans to stop this wonderful approach to natural health.

No matter what I say to you, some of you may still want to go it alone and that is fine as long as you have a track record for success. I've always been a bit of a doer and so I trust myself not to procrastinate to get the job done. Your job here is to get and stay healthy and perhaps even have some fun along the way.

I wasn't always so motivated. It is perfectly acceptable to need support, at least until you are consistent. Have you ever noticed that your success is only enjoyable once you've shared it with someone else? You get a promotion and you send an immediate text to your partner. You find out you're pregnant and you tell your mother. You book a holiday but not likely on your own. Success is always more tasty when shared. It's the same with your journey to health and well-being.

Sometimes it pays to ask for help. I recently had a dilemma about my mortgage. I wanted to get out of the mortgage, which would involve selling half of the property. I turned it over and over in my mind trying to determine how I could sell the domestic half of the property (there were legal problems with access). Months later, my partner Nic suggested I might think about selling the commercial space instead. Now, this might not seem like rocket science but I hadn't even considered the possibility of selling the commercial part of the property because I was so stuck on how to shift the domestic space. It took someone else to look on it with fresh eyes, to see something that now seems obvious.

A mentor, coach, teacher or group can see the things you often cannot see yourself. Daniel Priestley (entrepreneur and author) is fond of telling a story of mountains. Essentially the moral is that you cannot see the mountain you have climbed or how far you have come because you are standing on your own mountain. You only see the giant mountains in the distance that all the other people have succeeded in climbing. A mentor, coach, therapist or doctor can help you when you forget about the mountain you already stand upon and also hold you accountable for the actions you say you will take.

Don't be afraid to ask for help. The majority of healthcare practitioners (myself included) are doing what they do because they have suffered themselves. I love and teach posture and health because I know what it is to have posture-related health issues. Find someone to give you regular care and support. I often find that people use my online services to supplement their existing health and fitness regimes. Great! There is no room for professional arrogance. The more people helping you achieve your health goals, the better.

Address Your Lifestyle

Before you ask for help why not start by addressing your lifestyle. If I can be healthy, so can you! A close friend of mine is fond of saying, "You only live once." This is true. If it's only one time around, I want it to be an active *free* life. I certainly don't want to think about assisted care facilities and long days spent in front of the *idiot box** living out my golden years. How dreadful.

*TV [coined by Gerald Moore (aka Dad)]

If you've given little thought to how much alcohol you drink or what nutrition you provide your body or how often you choose to move your body, you may just find yourself at the age of 60 looking and feeling more like 80. I see this every day in practice and do you know what those 60-year-old clients of mine say? They don't say, "You only live once," but "Why didn't I start this years ago?" I really feel for these people, as the vast majority have started too late in life to reverse their premature ageing. Don't let this be you. Hangovers are not cool at 40.

Believe Yourself Healthy

When most of you think about lifestyle, you think about exercise and nutrition with little regard to your emotional well-being. I'm going to tell you something you can do to improve your health without actually *doing* anything! Now I've got your attention.

How do you explain that there are those of you who will reach the age of 75 and hit the ski slopes while others of you get moved into a nursing home to live out your golden years, assuming you all have the same access to food, exercise and healthcare services? Harvard psychologist Ellen Langer did an interesting study on hotel maids. She found the maids reported they did no regular exercise even though they cleaned 15 rooms a day, scrubbed toilets, pushed vacuums, pulled sheets and regularly walked several flights of stairs. Langer took several measures for fitness and discovered these women scored similar results to those with sedentary lifestyles. However, when Langer explained to the hotel maids all the daily exercise they were actually getting, those same women decreased their weight and body mass index and lowered their blood pressure by an incredible ten percent. The only thing that changed was their mindset.

If you believe you are healthy, your body behaves as a healthy body should. This is not to say, however, that you can trash your body, live on junk food and think it healthy – far from it. Langer tells us it is possible to use our thoughts to change our health. This is known as *mindfulness.* There has been some good research on how the mind affects health.

The Journal for Meditation and Meditation Research reports *mindfulness* as, 'the moment-to-moment attentional, unbiased observation of any phenomenon in order to perceive and to experience how it truly is, absent of emotional or intellectual distortion.' Mindfulness seems to concern our self-observations, thoughts, feelings, judgements, openness, insights, and understandings of our personal experiences. How often have you said to yourself, "I'm an idiot" or something equally negative? That is a perfect example of your mindfulness or lack thereof.

Mindfulness can be practised and one of my favourite mindfulness teachers is Eckhart Tolle. His book *The Power of Now* is a good read if you are a mindfulness beginner or try Osho's wonderfully accessible book *Joy: The Happiness That Comes From Within.*

So, Ellen Langer tells us that it's possible to change the health of our body with our thoughts but could it also be possible for our physical body to actually change the way we think? Well apparently it is.

Your Body Can Change Your Thoughts

A study on the science of confidence was conducted at Ohio State University. It found that the confidence of study participants was affected by whether the body posture they deliberately assumed was confident or not. Professor Richard Petty suggests that although most of us were taught that sitting up straight gives a good impression to other people, it turns out that our posture can also affect how we think about ourselves.

When the students held confident, upright posture they became more confident in their own thoughts. Those students that slouched and slumped were not even convinced by their own thoughts. The end result of this was that when students wrote positive thoughts about themselves (like their future job satisfaction and professional performance), they rated themselves more highly when in an upright posture because the upright posture led to confidence in their thoughts. This is exciting – your thoughts can change the health of your body (as Ellen Langer demonstrated with the hotel maids) and now it seems that your body position can change what you actually think about!

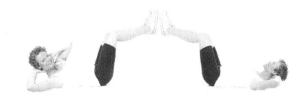

Don't Wait!

'For all the most important things, the timing always sucks. Waiting for a good time to quit your job? The stars will never align and the traffic lights of life will never all be green at the same time. The universe doesn't conspire against you, but it doesn't go out of its way to line up all the pins either. Conditions are never perfect. "Someday" is a disease that will take your dreams to the grave with you. If it's important to you and you want to do it "eventually," just do it and correct course along the way.' (Timothy Ferriss, author of *The 4 Hour Work Week)*

Relationships Suffer

I love to say to my youngish clients that "You are too damn young to feel so old." So many of you put off getting healthy, waiting for the signs and symptoms, aches and pains to become unbearable. Maybe you think starting next week is no different from starting today but I say that it is, because you cannot afford to put your health off for even just one more day. Your relationships suffer when you procrastinate with your health – the relationships with your partner, your kids, your work and, most importantly, with yourself.

Meet Donald

Donald is an amazing 90 years old and married to Jane aged 89. Donald embodies all that is agreeable in the world and it is obvious he has cultivated many good relationships. I see Donald regularly when he comes in for his spinal check-up. I love people like Donald; he is really living his life. He paints very well and goes to art class each week. He takes care of his wife (does all of the cooking and cleaning), dresses smartly (always sporting a tweed cap) and is never without a smile. I recently asked Donald what the secret to a long marriage is and he said, "Knowing when to shut up!" I am certain that it is his sense of humour, involvement with life and attention to his health that keeps him so jaunty.

Your Kids Suffer

Your health affects your family. I began recently with a new client. She came in with a history of lower back discomfort. When I took her medical history, it became clear to me that she had issues around food. Her entire family are obese and as a result she has spent her life in fear of being overweight. She is underweight and controls her food intake obsessively, often having nothing more than a small piece of toast in the mornings. She assures me that although she doesn't eat a good breakfast, she makes sure her children do.

So much of how we learn to eat and behave is a result of the patterns we learn from our parents. My sugar *addiction* was handed down from my family. Having dessert after every meal creates the scene for a lifetime of sugar cravings that I have to manage with great will-power and commitment to my own health.

Your children see all that you do; don't be fooled. They see and learn your emotions, your behaviours and your idiosyncrasies, whether you like it or not. It's not all bad so don't fret. It's your job to prepare your children for the challenges of life and that is what you do, even though it's not always glamorous or perfect. It is these family challenges that will help to create their adult strengths but don't fool yourself into thinking that your children will do as you say, not as you do. They will often do just as you do.

The biggest gift you can give to your children is a healthy habit. Teach them to love being active, to understand their bodies, to taste all varieties of food, to experience different cultures and express their creativity in the areas to which they naturally gravitate. I believe that the children I see in my practice have a definite advantage in life. They love jumping up on the tables and learning about their bodies. They enjoy the feeling of gentle touch and they ask me a million questions – *why, how, what, where, when* and *who*? They understand that health is something to celebrate. Health is fun and that is what they learn. What a great start in life.

Your Work Suffers

Good health gives you the energy and the opportunity to love the work that you do. A couple of years into private practice as a chiropractor, I completed some post-graduate training and earned a fellowship in the field of posture science. As a result of that training, a whole new world opened up for me and my work. I fell in love with posture and became slightly obsessed with correcting my own. I didn't always write; in fact I didn't even know how much I loved writing until I began blogging about posture. I do know that if you feel good in your body, you feel good in your life and as a result are more likely to choose work that you love.

Studies have associated manual, physical work and low job satisfaction with an increased risk of days off due to low back pain. If you focus on your stiff achy body all through your work day, it is very unlikely you will ever enjoy your work, regardless of the work that you do.

Recall the Ohio State University study that found study participants could convince their brains that their future job satisfaction and professional performance were likely to be good just by acquiring a more upright stance. Obviously, sitting up straight also gives a good impression to other people but, more importantly, if you sit up straight you end up convincing yourself by the posture you take. Good posture and good health go hand in hand. If you are already thinking that you would sit up straight if it didn't hurt so darn much, fear not. I will explain how you get past this hurdle shortly.

You Suffer

The most important relationship you have is the relationship with yourself. When you are not expressing your full health potential, the relationship you have with yourself suffers. There seems to be a plethora of chronic fatigue, fibromyalgia, depression and pain clinic referrals these days. Is this the *decade of syndromes*?

This isn't going to be a popular point of view but I'm afraid it is mine: I'm just not convinced by all these diagnoses. Now if you have been delivered one of these *sentences*, just keep reading. I see a lot of people who have been told they have chronic fatigue syndrome (Myalgia Encephalitis), fibromyalgia or depression and this is what else I see: Usually female (often mothers), 25-50, emotionally exhausted, often but certainly not always overweight, poor nutrition, history of anxiety and/or depression, dehydrated, *helpers* (more on this later), excess sugar intake, little exercise, regular use of pain medication and often waiting for a referral to the *pain clinic*.

These women (because they usually are women) come in *wearing* their pain. I can usually spot them a mile away and it is often referred to in medicine as their *sick role*. They like to tell their awful stories while embracing a rather characteristic slouching posture. They often cry and frequently apologise. They seem completely engulfed by their *labels – chronic fatigue, fibromyalgia* and/or *depression*.

This isn't meant to be harsh in any way. If this is a diagnosis (or as I prefer, *label*) you have been given and you find you are not getting any better, then you have nothing to lose by trying on what I have to say here. I often ask these women (once I have established trust) what they may be getting emotionally from remaining ill. This is often a very difficult area of investigation and not one I enter into lightly. I want to help women to learn to help themselves. I am a vitalist (whole body practitioner) and I truly believe these women have everything within themselves to heal, despite their *label*.

Whatever your label or health concerns, consider the possibility that there may be a *pay-off* for remaining unwell.

Who would choose to be sick? I believe that many would and do. Sickness may provide something that is lacking for many of you. You may need to dig deeply and open yourself up to some emotional pain but it will be worth it so try it on. What, if anything, do you think you get from staying ill? Let me give you an example from my own life.

I have a tendency, from time to time, to experience sadness. I call it being *flat*. I'm sure I could have had a diagnosis or label of depression several times over had I seen a medical doctor over the years. Instead I choose to accept these fluctuations as normal. Do I like it? No way! Is it worse if I give it a label and look for an external cause or solution that is out of my control? Definitely!

When you have a personality like I do, the lows come with the highs, as day comes with night, black with white and hot with cold. I am quite certain I would not appreciate the great passions and excitement of my life if I did not know my sadness intimately. Sometimes when I am *flat*, I see that I could easily use this to remain inactive – preventing my ongoing growth as a Posture Doctor, chiropractor, businesswoman, partner, friend, daughter and creator. Occasionally, I do use it. I see my flatness as my body's way of giving me a mandatory break from the incessant hive of brain activity. My pay-off for being sad is that I don't have to *go for it,* just in case it doesn't work out. Do you recognise this in you?

There may be many other types of pay-offs. Perhaps you get attention from a distracted spouse, or you get to control things or maybe you get to experience being loved and cared for. I encourage you to look openly to recognise your own pay-offs. Don't be surprised if this feels like too large a task. Some of you may find therapy a necessary part of your healing and health.

Chronic Fatigue Syndrome

I am uncomfortable with the diagnosis of chronic fatigue syndrome because of the lack of scientific understanding of the cause and the limited approach to helpful treatment (often only medication). There are so many factors that are involved with chronic fatigue that I feel it is unfair to label someone with this *sentence* until a reasonable effort has been made to address each issue.

When dealing with fatigue I address sleep habits, nutrition (skipping breakfast, caffeine, sugar, fruit and vegetables, quality of food and hydration), medication use, smoking and alcohol, posture, emotional support, work satisfaction and activity levels. There is absolutely no way that someone can feel alive and vibrant when these factors have not been addressed. This isn't a quick process but one that I believe delivers lasting, lifelong results.

Fibromyalgia

I am weary of labelling my patients with the diagnosis of fibromyalgia. I find most of the people who have been given this as a diagnosis have been given it incorrectly, regardless of whether or not it is a valid condition. The actual process of presenting fibromyalgia as a diagnosis involves a physical examination. If you have been given this *label* without a physical examination you have every right to question its validity. The American College of Rheumatology has set criteria for the diagnosis: Pain in 11 of 18 tender sites, in a patient with pain for at least three months. The tender points are found in specific locations and must be on both sides of the body and above and below the waist. I have **never** seen a new client who has been given the diagnosis of fibromyalgia by another health professional who was examined as per the American College guidelines.

I approach all clients who have been given *labels* just as I would any other person that I examine and treat. I assess their physical, chemical and emotional well-being. I address the physical (past traumas and exercise) with chiropractic *adjustments* along with posture exercises and corrective rehabilitation. I address the chemical (food and drink they consume, toxins, environment) with nutrition and lifestyle advice. I address the emotional through breathing, lifestyle and sometimes a referral for emotional support, if appropriate.

Depression

Depression, formerly melancholia, has a long history indeed. Melancholia (*melas*, 'black' and *khole*, 'bile') was derived from ancient Greek. Hippocrates described it as 'fears and despondencies, if they last a long time'. Robert Burton, 17th century English scholar, suggests in his book *The Anatomy of Melancholy*, that 'melancholy could be combated with a healthy diet, sufficient sleep, music, and "meaningful work", along with talking about the problem with a friend'. This advice seems to have stood the test of time.

The term melancholia was used until the term *depression* (from the Latin verb 'to press down') gained popularity in the 16th century and began appearing in medical dictionaries in the mid 1800s. Aristotle had used the term melancholia as an associated hazard of contemplation and creativity. I love this explanation and it is one I believe captures my own periods of flatness.

It was Freud who popularised the view of internal and external types of depression but this was and is largely debated, depending on the psychodynamic theory to which you subscribe. Freud emphasised our life's experiences as predisposing factors.

In the mid-20th century it was theorised that depression was caused by chemical imbalances in the brain. People seem almost charmed into talking about their 'chemical imbalance' and that *imbalance* is often worn like a label. I certainly don't deny the existence of such an imbalance but it is this very imbalance that seems to be interpreted as a permanent fixture without any chance of rebalancing.

Mechanists (recall the opposite of *vitalist*) approach this chemical imbalance by using an *outside-in* approach. Such an approach is, more often than not, medication. The medication is not without its share of controversy. Today, there is criticism of the ever-expanding definition of depression and how it may relate to the development and promotion of antidepressants.

SSRIs or selective serotonin re-uptake inhibitors are used in depression to allow an increase in cellular serotonin (the hormone related to several body processes, including mood). How effective these drugs are in the *treatment* of depression has been disputed. The reported side effects have included nausea, headache, fatigue, insomnia, suicidal thoughts and increased **risk of depression** to name but a few.

There is some very encouraging **vitalistic** research on depression. Some studies have shown that daily walking is at least as effective, if not better than some antidepressant medication and there is evidence to suggest that people get better over time with or without the use of drugs. I can certainly see that sometimes medication may play a short-term role in *sick-care*, but more often than not I see young women and men left taking antidepressants for years and years, creating long-term dependence.

More recently, depression has been considered genetic and thus inevitable but epigeneticists like Dr Bruce Lipton would argue that our genes are merely blueprints that can be changed. He explains that a gene may suggest you have a predisposition to something but that predisposition (whether or not the gene gets *turned on)* is down to the physical, chemical and emotional environment in which you bathe your genes.

Recall that a true vitalistic approach to health care looks at the whole person. When dealing with depression, vitalism is key. A vitalistic healthcare provider will look at your physical, chemical and emotional environment and approach your illness by addressing all three. If these three elements are addressed, I believe that depression can be eased in many cases, without the need for dangerous, addictive medication. If you think you may have depression, make sure you have the support of a qualified vitalistic healthcare practitioner. You should always make decisions about your antidepressant medication alongside your doctor.

Survive Or Thrive?

Do you want to survive life or would you prefer to truly thrive? I choose the latter. When did getting up in the morning become such a chore? When did we stop skipping down the pavement without feeling silly? When did we start caring so much about what everyone else thinks? Is this what it is to be an adult? If so, I'm not playing!

Some of my most cherished memories are from my childhood and also the past ten years of my life. I have vivid memories of whole days spent outdoors – swimming in the river, constructing roadways in my sandbox, climbing trees, twirling on my merry-go-round (my father put one in our back garden), ice skating and running, running and more running. I had boundless energy and enthusiasm for life. Oh, there were family arguments, school tests and getting teased, but these memories have faded away and what remains is the imprint of a happy childhood. I was thriving.

Something happens along the way. It is as if life begins to weigh us down – university exams, the pressure of deciding on *the one thing* we want to do when we grow up, paying bills, broken hearts and other responsibilities take over. Then one day you find you are trapped in a mediocre job with a mediocre relationship, a mortgage, kids and the time you spend waiting between holidays.

I hope that, for many of you, life is better than the picture I've painted. Perhaps those of you reading this book are the very ones who refuse to accept *survival* as enough. Good for you! If there is one thing that I am absolutely certain of, it is that **your life is for living**! You must thrive and you cannot thrive and do the things you'd love to do with an exhausted, unfit body. Remember Timothy Ferriss's admonishment: 'Someday is a disease that will take your dreams to the grave with you ... just do it and correct course along the way.' Start today!

Conditions Related To Bad Posture

Your posture is what everybody looks at when they see you. One medical study in The American Journal of Pain Management related: 'Spine pain, headache, mood, blood pressure, pulse and lung capacity' among the 'functions most easily influenced by posture'. Another study in the Journal of the American Geriatric Society suggested that 'older men and women with hyperkyphotic posture have higher mortality rates'.

In 2005, a study in the journal *Spine* suggested: 'All measures of health showed poorer scores as forward head and body posture increased'. In other words, those with forward head posture have a lower health status. In 2007, the Archives of Internal Medicine reported that 'height loss was associated with a 42% increased risk of coronary events such as heart attacks'. There is also plenty of anecdotal evidence to suggest that there are many conditions caused by bad posture:

- *Chronic fatigue syndrome*
- *Headaches*
- *Dizziness*
- *Nasal congestion*
- *Asthma*
- *Palpitations*
- *Reflux (stomach acid)*
- *Constipation*
- *High blood pressure*

There is enough evidence to strongly suggest that you need to begin addressing your posture today. Don't wait for your symptoms before beginning a programme of correction because your relationships with your children, work and ultimately yourself will suffer. You have the choice – you can survive or, if you start today, you may actually begin to thrive and what a life that will be! Read on and I will teach you how!

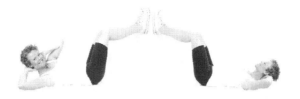

CHAPTER SEVEN

Avoid Premature Ageing

Nobody likes to feel old, especially those of you feeling old at just 30 or 40. No thank you! You need to understand what is happening and how you can prevent it. Morning stiffness is a sign of *sarcopenia*. If you are over 25, sarcopenia (flesh loss) has already begun. Yikes, sounds scary but it's not really. Sarcopenia is the degenerative loss of skeletal muscle mass and strength associated with ageing. The amount of sarcopenia depends on how regular and lifelong your exercise has been.

Sarcopenia is a real concern because of society's diminishing physical activity (think internet) and increasing longevity. We're living too darn long. Sarcopenia may progress to the point where an older person loses the ability to live independently as this condition is linked with poor balance, walking speed, falls and broken bones. Sarcopenia results in a significant amount of frailty in the elderly. Don't worry, you are going to learn what you need to do.

It's Not Your Age

'Is this normal for my age?' These words drive me to utter distraction. It's not your age! If having wear in your joints was normal for your age, you'd see it evenly distributed throughout all of your joints, but you don't. You see it in your hip (that short left leg), or your knee (the one you fell on ten years ago), or your shoulder (the collar bone fracture?). Do you see? The *wear and tear* in your body has to do with your lifetime of physical, chemical and emotional stress and not some random act of chance, called *age*.

The process of *wear and tear* began long before the aches and pains that you now experience – so it really wasn't that box you lifted or the sneeze or even the gardening. Yes, these things aggravated your body but, believe me, the problem was waiting for an excuse to show itself and now it has.

The Arthritis Con

I am going to set the record straight here and call a spade a spade. *Wear and tear* is just the non-scary way of saying *osteoarthritis*. There, I've said it. My clients say to me, "My doctor said I have *wear and tear* in my neck but I don't think it's arthritis." I'm sorry to say it to you, but *wear and tear* is arthritis. This is where I think the confusion lies.

When most of you think of arthritis, you think of granny's hunched back. There are many different types of arthritis, many more than the two I'll discuss here. One type of arthritis is caused by your own immune dysfunction – your body attacking itself. One example of this type of arthritis is rheumatoid arthritis. This type of arthritis more commonly begins at a younger age and often leaves sufferers with disfigured joints.

Rheumatoid

Often joint pain is referred to as *rheumatism*, from the ancient Greek '*rheum*' meaning *humour* and *discharge.* Humour is from the Hippocratic theory of disease and illness arising from one of the four humours (blood, bile, yellow bile and phlegm). If you have joint pain you may be referred to a rheumatologist who specialises in the diagnosis and treatment of arthritis and related conditions. If you have one of the arthridities caused by your own immune system, a blood test will usually diagnose this.

Osteo

Blood tests aren't usually taken to diagnose osteoarthritis. *Osteo* (meaning bone) arthritis can be diagnosed easily by x-ray. A simple x-ray shows the bones and the spaces between the bones where the cartilage is. Worn cartilage, bone spurs, rough joint surfaces can all be seen on x-ray and this is what constitutes osteoarthritis. Because you usually do not start to feel the effects of these worn joint surfaces until some time into your 30s, 40s or 50s, osteoarthritis is thought of as an older person's arthritis. Personally, I would prefer it if practitioners stopped telling people, 'It's normal for your age' because what is seen in one 30-, 40-, 50- or 80-year-old is largely variable and simply isn't down to your age as such.

How To Stay Motivated

'It's not what you are that holds you back;
it's what you think you are not.'

Denis Waitley

By the time most of you begin having signs and symptoms (morning stiffness, aches, pains and creaking) the osteoarthritis has already begun. It is for this reason I suggest you find the motivation you need to start now. I hear you: 'It's too much like hard work'; 'It's going to take too long'; 'I've already tried everything'; 'It's not a major problem really.' Sound familiar?

You put things off in life because the pain isn't painful enough. You know you want to cut down on your drinking but you like it, right? Some people will stop drinking only when it becomes a measurably painful activity (in other words when they admit they are alcoholics). When do people really get serious about quitting smoking? When that life sentence of a diagnosis is handed out – **cancer**! When do people really start living life? When they are told they have six months to live.

I know these are extreme examples but I really want you to get it. There is no magic cure – it must come from you. If you keep on doing what you are doing (or not doing) you will likely start to experience the signs and symptoms of premature ageing. If only my *older* clients (I'm only talking 50-60 years here) could speak to you, they would say they wish they had started sooner. If you fail to begin, you have a much greater chance of developing a chronic problem. Don't delay, you will only regret it.

What will it take to get you motivated enough to take on your health? Are you waiting for it to be painful enough? Are you waiting for the joint pain to be unbearable? Your family relationships to suffer? Your self-esteem to hit rock bottom? We are funny things we humans. I know that physical pain is a great motivator but you'd best find something a little more emotionally relevant if you want to keep at it, because if you don't you will give up when the pain is gone and you find yourself back at square one a few months later.

The best way to stay motivated with anything in your life is to become really clear about **why** you want to do it. Here is an example from my own life. What has me indoors, at my computer, writing this book on a beautiful sunny day, when I could be down on Brighton beach? Do I feel hard done by? No. Do I long for the beach? No. Is there something else I'd rather be doing? NO! If those answers were yes, I'd never finish this book. I'm going to finish this book because I know *why* I'm writing it.

I'm not talking about wishy-washy *whys* either – like it's fun and cool to be an author and make some money. Those may be valid reasons but they aren't going to tug at my emotions and keep me writing. Really dig deep for your *whys*. My *whys* for this book are these: To become well known as an expert in posture correction, to reach people in countries on every continent, to speak about health and posture internationally and to one day live back in Canada on my favourite lake (probably writing more books). The more specific you can be, the more likely you are to stick with your health commitments.

Don't make your goals, *to quit smoking* or *to lose weight* – dig deep. Maybe you want to regain powerful lungs so you can play with your kids for longer than five minutes. Perhaps you want to get a body you'd feel sexy in, so you could begin salsa classes. Maybe you've always wanted your own vegetable garden or you dream of lying on a beach in South America for a one-month luxury holiday. Whatever it is that turns you on, be specific and you are more likely to succeed. Ask yourself: "If I couldn't fail, what would I do?"

Stop Brain Fog

One sign of premature ageing is what I like to call *brain fog*. Good posture imparts massive health benefit, allowing for full lung expansion and diaphragm movement, which improves breathing. Better breathing means more oxygen to the lungs and body tissues, including the brain. When you have poor posture, you reduce your vital lung capacity by up to 30%!

Good oxygen levels can provide relief from headache and migraine, stress, fatigue, muscle cramps, jet lag, hangovers and general aches and pains. Oxygen speeds up recovery from physical exertion, improves metabolism and digestion and improves your sleep and skin tone. Oxygen can heighten your concentration, alertness and energy levels and ultimately reduce *brain fog*.

Your lung capacity dictates how much oxygen your lungs can take in when you breathe. If you think about oxygen as food for your brain, it is not hard to understand the concept of *brain fog*. My patients often describe having a *muzzy head*, feeling tired, having low energy or generally feeling a bit spaced out.

HEALTHY TIP

- *Open windows daily and sleep with an open window*

- *Drink more water – water contains oxygen (drink enough so your urine is clear)*

- *Drink one glass of water for every cup of tea or coffee (caffeine dehydrates)*

- *Use plants to reduce indoor air pollution and increase oxygen (two plants per 100 ft^2)*

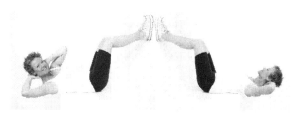

CHAPTER EIGHT

What About My Pain?

It's never too late to start getting healthy but you mustn't leave it for even one more day. Inactivity rapidly de-conditions your body. The elastic band that isn't stretched dries up and breaks. You mustn't wait for the pain to begin. In this chapter I will teach you to trust your body to heal and the secret to lowering your pain threshold. You will learn the three factors needed to determine your body's 'real age' and how to be certain you have healthy strong bones. Ready?

Is It Too Late For Me?

'I should have come to see you years ago.' These are the words I hear almost daily in practice. I too wish that I had had chiropractic treatment when I was a child. As it turns out, I took myself to a chiropractor in my early 20s. Sadly for me, I'd stopped growing, had forward head posture and a right *leg length deficiency* that has caused my lower back much aggravation over the years. I believe that my posture and lower back health would have been very different had I seen a chiropractor and addressed my posture before I had finished growing.

It is **never** too late to get support and help for your body but so much more can be done if you do not wait until the signs and symptoms begin. Often by this time you already have arthritis and premature ageing.

If you have symptoms, you need help and many of you who don't have symptoms need to *start now* before chronic problems begin. Are you gearing up to start getting healthy a few months from now, when you have the time? Don't! Have you ever noticed how hard it is to get to the gym after work even though you had great intentions when you woke up in the morning? Morning is not the best time to exercise in terms of your body's preparation, but realistically morning is best for most of us because it's the only time we'll do it.

I exercise every morning because if I didn't do it then, it wouldn't happen and not because I don't enjoy it, but because I'd be too tired to do it. This isn't an argument for the best time for exercise but for recognising that when we future date the beginning of something as important as exercise, we tell our brains that other things matter more to us than our health. They must not! We only go around once in life (as far as I know anyway) and I'm certain we all want our latter years to be active and not ticking away in a nursing home with premature ageing and bedpans.

Don't Wait For The Pain

This is how some of you think: 'I'll wait until I need it.' By *need it* you most certainly mean when the symptoms get bad enough you can't take it any more. Let's apply this same approach to your car. I think it is fair to say that most of us have our cars serviced regularly. Do you only have your car serviced when it is spluttering along the roadside or after the oil light has been on for several weeks? Do you put a piece of tape over the oil light? Seems crazy, right? That is what you do with your bodies. You take pills to mask the pain and you wait and wait and wait. When you finally can't stand it any more, you come and see me and wonder why it takes so long to get well. Good grief.

If you are waiting for the pain to show itself before you do something about your health, then don't worry, it's coming. That is one thing that I am absolutely certain of. By the time the pain begins, your problems have often become chronic and are more difficult to address and treat. I understand that pain is a great motivator but do yourself a massive favour and don't wait. Start now!

What Is Pain?

I'm also surprised to find out how poorly people are able to describe their pain. "How would you describe your headache?" I ask them, to which I'm often given an, "It hurts," or "It's just painful, really painful." When I step back and consider why this is, I recognise that pain is very poorly understood by most people who have not spent any time studying science or the human body (so most people, really). When you tell me that your arm hurts, I understand that most of you believe the pain (that very *real* thing) is actually in your arm.

When I was explaining pain to my creative *other* one day, I explained that arm pain isn't in the arm. I got an expression that basically said, 'yeah right.' I went on to explain: The nerve endings that communicate pain to the brain (nocicepetors) are located in the arm but the actual experience of pain is in the head. So the next time you are being judged an emotional wreck and told, "It's all in your head," you can turn around and say, "I know it is!"

This may be a strange concept for some of you. The next time you have pain, remember that pain isn't bad. Your pain is simply the activation of those specialised nerves called nociceptors. These nerves respond to changes in your environment (temperature, mechanical and chemical changes) and then send signals to your brain and spinal cord so you can take appropriate action. If you put your hand near something hot, your nociceptors for temperature fire off, sending a message to your spinal cord which then sends a message back to your hand and you move it away from the potentially dangerous stimulant (the hot burner).

I'm sure you recognise that this is a good process. You want to know when things are hot so you don't get burned.

Similarly, you want to understand what your body is communicating when it has pain. The last thing you want to do is suppress your body – in a sense, shutting it up. What is your body saying? Get interested. Be fascinated by your wonderfully functioning body. What is your headache saying? *Drink some water, move your body, take a break, I have a virus, there are chemicals in this space, my posture needs attention, I'm hungry.*

HEALTHY TIP

You can start altering your relationship to pain by learning to listen and understand all the different speakings from your marvellous body. When you need to use the toilet, go and use the toilet straight away; don't wait and don't just finish writing that last email. When you are hungry, stop what you are doing and get something to eat; don't wait. When you are sluggish, get some fresh air; don't wait. When you are tired at night, go to bed and don't just sit and watch one more programme like a zombie. I too am guilty of ignoring my body but these days I make a real effort to listen to its many communications. Try this and notice how often you ignore your body.

Suppressing Your Pain

Another favourite approach to dealing with pain is to medicate. One thing I say to my patients is this: "Do you think that your painkiller knows how to find the headache (or back pain, or arm pain)?" My question to you is: "Do you think perhaps that pill you take affects your whole body or does it just target the problem area?" Of course that pill affects your whole body. That is the main problem with medication – that and all the chemicals *we* are putting into our bodies and the havoc they cause.

Now back to the oil light on your car. The light glows red and you think to yourself, 'the car definitely shouldn't be doing this'. Then you take a piece of black electrical tape and cover over the red light. You feel better now that you can't see the red light – can't see the light, so the problem is gone. Ah, but of course the problem is not gone, it has only been masked, hidden and forgotten. How long do you think your car will keep running until you actually have to address the problem? Eventually the car will break down and oh boy, don't you wish you had just put the oil in the tank earlier? Now you have a huge repair bill. Darn it! Luckily, you can always buy a new car. Not so lucky with your body though. You only get one. Suppressing and ignoring your body's messages (your aches and pains) will only lead to trouble.

Your Pain Threshold?

Do you think that you have a high pain threshold? In other words if somebody says, "I thought I was dying," when they have a headache, are you more likely to say, "It was pretty bad, but it didn't stop me doing anything"? I see a huge variation in pain threshold with my clients. I like to use a simple pain scale. I ask them to rate their pain on a scale of one to ten with ten being the worst pain they have experienced in their lives. I am always shocked when a client says to me, "The pain isn't that bad, maybe a seven." Wow! A seven to me is severe pain.

There is increasing evidence to suggest that medicating our pain lowers our pain threshold over time. So, much like the alcoholic who now needs six drinks to get a buzz when it used to take only three, you find yourself needing a lot more pain medication to deal with your headache. Perhaps you aren't even sure if those pills make any difference but you habitually take them.

One of my clients told me he still *needs* to carry his pain medication with him everywhere he goes. If he doesn't have it with him, his worry creates a tension headache. Medication may make your body so unable to fend for itself that a painful stimulus which in the past would have had you say 'ouch' now has you scream bloody murder. This has to stop. Stop shutting your body up. Let it learn to heal itself. Learn to trust your body to heal and you will find that one day your pain is no longer an issue.

When you first begin this process, it will be challenging. If you are used to reaching for the painkillers your brain will scream at you to take them. You may even hear yourself saying, "I tried for a while but then I had to take something." Watch these words closely: *had to*. You rarely *have to* do anything, unless someone is forcing a pill down your throat. You really need to see that it is your choice whether or not to medicate your pain.

Lower your pain threshold

It takes about a month before the pain pill habit becomes an un-habit and eventually (even if you believe it is not possible) you won't even think about taking something, you will just naturally ask yourself what your body needs. I promise you, this can happen. For many years I regularly took aspirin for my headaches and now it has been over 15 years without **any** form of medication. What do I do when I get a headache (yes, sometimes a healthy body gets a headache)? I take the pain. The good news is that after months and years of not medicating, the intensity of your pain becomes very manageable. These days if I get a headache, it scores no higher than about a one or two out of ten in severity. In essence, I have learned to lower my pain threshold and so can you!

HEALTHY
TIP

Do you know why rubbing your stubbed toe makes it feel better? It confuses your brain's pain signals and gives it something else to think about. What that means is that your current pain threshold can be lowered by:

- *Listening to your pain and other body signals (what is your body trying to tell you?)*

- *Breaking the pain medication habit*

- *Distracting your brain (rub the sore spot, do a puzzle, or dust off that old hula-hoop)*

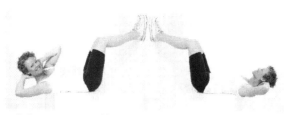

CHAPTER NINE

How Well Are You Ageing?

It is never too late to begin to get healthy but every day that you wait, your body is ageing in ways that are often irreversible. There is a difference between your chronological and physiological age. Your chronological age is the number of years you have been alive whilst your physiological age is the real age of your body. There is some debate as to what markers you should use to determine your physiological age and there are some interesting online tests you can take. Without getting too scientific, there are some good clues as to your physiological age.

The Three Markers Of Age

Jamie Timmons, Professor of Ageing Biology at Birmingham University, believes the three most relevant markers for how well you age physiologically are:

- *Insulin sensitivity*
- *Aerobic fitness*
- *Genetics*

Insulin is a protein hormone that removes the sugar*
from your blood. When your body becomes ineffective at
removing sugars, you develop diabetes. This marker for
ageing will be strongly related to your **nutritional habits**.

*Glucose or sugar comes from the food we eat such as fruit, bread,
pasta and other carbohydrates. These foods are broken down into
sugar and then absorbed into the bloodstream.

Aerobic fitness is all about how good your heart and
lungs are at getting oxygen into the body. The important
measure here is your vital lung capacity. Aerobic fitness
is affected by the frequency and type of exercise you take
and also **strongly associated** with your body posture.
Dr Rene Cailliet, doctor of musculo-skeletal medicine,
reminds us that poor posture (particularly slouching) can
reduce your vital lung capacity by 30%!

People respond to exercise in very different ways, as the
Heritage Family Study explains. The study suggests that
the third marker for ageing – genetics – can be thought
of in terms of the variation in your muscular DNA. It
reasons that some people will be *non-responders* when it
comes to exercise and this might explain why some people
seem to exercise without seeing any obvious results (like
weight loss). Luckily for most, this is the exception, not the
rule. Recall also Dr Bruce Lipton's field of epigenetics that
reminds us that our genetic expression can be influenced
by our physical, chemical and emotional environments.
No longer are we victims of our genetics!

How Old Are Your Bones?

The age of your bones may tell you a lot about how well your body and skeleton will age. Will you be active at 80? The health of your bones is based on what you feed your body, your hormones, when menopause occurs, the physical traumas your body has sustained and the amount and type of exercise you have had over your lifetime. All of these factors determine your *peak bone mass.*

Your skeleton completely replaces itself every seven years and for children it is every two years. Your bones are living tissue and old bone is continually replaced by new. During childhood you deposit much more new bone than you lose so your skeleton grows in length and density. By the time you turn 18-21, you will have gained roughly 90% of your peak bone mass and this is why youth is the best time to invest in making strong bones through exercise. Get your kids off Facebook!

Your Peak Bone Mass

Your bone mass is the amount of bone tissue in your skeleton and this continues to build up to its maximum density by age 30. This is why putting off exercise for even just one more day is too long. During your menopausal years (usually three to five years) you will lose about 15% from your peak bone mass. If your peak mass was low to begin with, you may be vulnerable to weak bones and osteoporosis. Men do not have the same bone loss with age as women do, because they do not have a rapid decline in their hormone levels. This helps to protect men from osteoporosis.

Your peak bone mass is the total density of your bones prior to the 15% loss (for women) at menopause. If your peak bone mass was relatively high before the inevitable loss and your current lifestyle supports bone maintenance, then your bones will likely stand you in good stead for your *golden years.* If however your peak bone mass was low at 30 and your lifestyle is poor now, then you are more vulnerable to premature ageing through bone loss.

Up to age 30	Lifestyle now
high peak bone mass	+ low rate bone loss = **strong bones**
low peak bone mass	+ high rate bone loss = **weak bones**

Are You At Risk?

I've created a bone mass quiz based on many of the questions I would ask you if you came to see me in practice. This quiz is only a guide and cannot replace the accuracy of an actual bone mineral density scan. If you are concerned by your score, then you can discuss this with your doctor and perhaps request a bone scan privately if not available to you through your National Health Service. This test is designed for those of you who have yet to reach menopause.

Scoring:

take the indicated points for each **YES** *and
record* **zero points** *for each* **NO.**

1 *Were you overweight as a child?
(over 7lbs)* **YES** *(1 point)*

2 *Were you an active child?* **YES** *(-1 point)*

3 *Have you ever broken your leg or wrist?* **YES** *(1 point)*

4 *Is there any family history of joint
replacements? (knees, hips)* **YES** *(1 point)*

5 *Do you wake up stiff in the mornings?
(at least once a week)* **YES** *(1 point)*

6 *Do you have a desk job?* **YES** *(1 point)*

7 *Do you smoke?* **YES** *(2 points)*

8 *Do you drink fizzy or sugary drinks?* **YES** *(1 point)*

9 *Do you take regular exercise?
(more than twice a week)* **YES** *(-2 points)*

10 *Have you ever fallen from a height?
(horse, stairs, tree)* **YES** *(1 point)*

11 *Are you overweight? (over 10 pounds)* **YES** *(1 point)*

12 *Do you take caffeine?
(more than 2 tea or 1 coffee each day)* **YES** *(1 point)*

13 *Do you use any medication?
(more than once a month)* **YES** *(1 point)*

14 *Do you have a noticeable fatty
neck lump?* **YES** *(1 point)*

CONTINUED OVER ▶

15 *Have you had ongoing menstrual problems?*   **YES** *(2 points)*

16 *Have you had a hysterectomy?*   **YES** *(3 points)*

17 *Do you eat fruit and vegetables? (at least three portions a day)*   **YES** *(-1 point*

18 *Do you drink alcohol? (more than three drinks a week)*   **YES** *(1 point)*

19 *Have you had breast cancer or have a strong family history of it?*   **YES** *(3 points)*

20 *Have you taken long-term steroids? **   **YES** *(3 points)*

* Steroid medications (like those used for asthma and other acute inflammation), in high dose and with prolonged use, can cause growth suppression. Steroids decrease the amount of new bone formation. This may be crucial when considering steroids for a child. Steroids also increase the breakdown of bone and decrease the absorption of calcium from food. It is advisable to have regular bone scans to assess the strength of your bones if you are at risk (menopausal, underweight, previous fractures, poor nutrition, strong family history, sedentary, smoker, radiation treatment, hysterectomy).

Score Totals -

0-5
(low to slight risk – some lifestyle changes are advisable)

6-10
(at risk – you would benefit from a physical examination)

11-17
(moderate risk – a bone scan should be discussed with your healthcare provider)

18-25
(high risk – consider having a bone scan even if you have to pay privately)

Three factors need to be considered for healthy strong bones:

1 Your Hormones

Oestrogen has a protective effect on your bones so if you began menstruating late (due to very high activity levels and low body weight) and you begin menopause early, you may be at higher risk of having weak bones.

2 How Acid Is Your Diet?

Some of you may be surprised to learn that the food and drink you regularly consume may be weakening your bones. Wheat, strong cheese, caffeine (and cigarettes), sugar, red meat, fizzy drinks and alcohol are all acidic. Our blood is slightly alkaline (the opposite pH to acid) and that is where your body prefers to be. In order to balance the acidity of these foods, your body leaches calcium from your bones to offset the acidic pH. You can Google *alkaline foods* to get an idea of the types of foods that will help to keep your bones strong.

To maintain strong bones you also need a good supply of calcium and, contrary to popular belief, dairy isn't the best source. Dairy is on the acidic side of the food chart and it is also not the easiest form of calcium to absorb. You can get a good supply of calcium from dark leafy vegetables, beans and peas, grains, seafood and seeds.

You also need vitamin D to absorb calcium and vitamin D is made through skin exposure to the sun. Think of the sun as food for your bones. Sunlight stimulates the production of vitamin D so you need at least 20 minutes outdoors every day without sun screen.

Fish oils are a perfect source of vitamin D, provided you know that your source of fish isn't full of mercury. This is the one supplement I think we all need. I take a teaspoon a day of high quality fish oils (don't go budget here). Get the best quality fish oils you can afford.

3 Exercise And Posture

You hear it all the time but weight-bearing exercise is absolutely crucial to strong bones and to maintain your existing bone mass. Riding a bike and swimming are great for your heart but they are weightless so don't help your bones as such. Fast paced walking (with good arm swing), hiking, tennis, running if you are under 35, weight-lifting, pilates, yoga, martial arts and dancing are all good choices.

Your posture is crucial to the health of your bones. If your body is out of its symmetrical alignment, there is uneven pressure and stress on your joints and this can lead to wear and tear (osteoarthritis) in those joints.

HEALTHY
TIP

Eat some seeds. You will need sesame seeds, pumpkin seeds, sunflower seeds and linseeds (aka flaxseed). Keep them in a glass sealed jar in the fridge. Use a small coffee grinder (these aren't expensive) and grind a tablespoon of seeds each day. Add them to salads, porridge, cereals, greens, rice, soup or dry roast in a frying pan for an easy crunchy snack. Seeds are a great source of calcium and they have the good fats needed for a healthy heart, brain, joints and glowing skin!

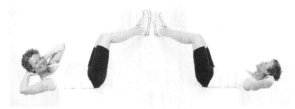

CHAPTER TEN

Start To Heal Your Posture

'We are what we repeatedly do.
Excellence, then, is not an act, but a habit.'

Aristotle

Inactivity is a slow killer. You can sit too much and you can even sleep too much. Getting outside, getting active has the potential to take years off you. But I don't mean you need to start training for the New York Marathon. You can start changing your body with only your thoughts and then begin to get healthy and correct your posture with just eight minutes' exercise a day!

Step 1 (De-clutter Your Brain)

Do you have a light bulb in your house that needs changing? How about a broken electrical appliance? Something to get rid of, an unpaid bill, plants to water, dishes to clean, a load of washing that needs doing? How many times over how many days, weeks or months have you looked at that pile of papers? Do you know that your *unfinished business* takes up valuable mental, emotional and physical energy – energy that could free you to take on something meaningful, like correcting your posture and getting healthy?

My father – a wise pain-in-the-butt! he was – used to look at my bedroom (the bomb site) and say to me, "How can you think straight in here? Cluttered desk, cluttered mind!" He was right and, darn it, I swore never to let that happen.

My partner Nic is a creative sort and has been de-cluttering since we met. I see how a cluttered environment weighs heavily on one so talented and it frustrates me to see such untapped creative potential. Is this you? Even just a bit? I used to be quite a messy child and shared a room with my little sister. I slept late and threw my clothes on the floor – normal kid stuff – but something changed along the way.

Since the end of university I have noticed that I have simplified my life. I have less and less *stuff* and I have less need to have big things in my life. My point here is simple: I fill my life with the good *stuff*. I have time to do the work that I love, like writing this book. I have time for daily exercise. I have time for my relationships and I have time to do nothing (chill-out time). Oh, and I still have time to get overwhelmed, stressed and frustrated but I think that is part of a healthy existence.

If you want room in your life to change your health, you need room in your life. It is time to clear the decks. If you need help, ask for it. I've been offering to help Nic for two years but I don't recommend getting your significant other to help you de-clutter your life. Recipe for disaster! There are people who specialise in this line of work and can help you. Google them. Start now. Start today!

Step 2 (Think Yourself Healthy)

Exercise early in life hard-wires your brain to experience exercise as a *normal* behaviour. If you have somehow managed to avoid exercise your whole life, you may be one of a growing minority who say they 'hate it'. If you are adamant that you do, I am going to challenge that belief. I'm sure only very few of you actually 'hate it' and most likely because it makes you short of breath, ache or feel embarrassed about your body or any number of valid reasons. But, and this is a really *big butt* (pun definitely intended), it doesn't have to be like this.

First things first. Before you get yourself a fit body, you have to stop with the negativity if you want to get exercising, correct your posture and get healthy. Lose the word *hate* for good. It's such a nasty, strong word anyway. Can you imagine if you constantly said to yourself *I hate kissing* and then tried to attract a mate? If you *hate* exercise, you'll never correct your posture. So lose *hate* from your vocabulary.

To begin with, it doesn't even matter if you believe the words that you say to yourself. Apparently your subconscious mind cannot tell the difference between real and imagined. That is why you jump when you watch a scary movie. Your rational mind knows the scary man is an actor but your subconscious brain has you jump out of your skin. The theory goes that you can implant suggestions into your mind to effect permanent change. Simply start with some positive words to describe your relationship to your body, exercise and health.

HEALTHY TIP

Write down the negative words (OLD TALK) you use when you talk about exercising your body

Next, write out some **NEW TALK** *to describe your exercising body*

Now choose a date to start using the new talk

Ask for help (tell friends and family to point out whenever you revert to the old talk)

Write the new talk on your bathroom mirror (use non-permanent marker)

Commit to practising the new talk for 30 days

e.g. OLD TALK	*I hate exercise*	
NEW TALK	I'm gettin' me a new bod	
e.g. OLD TALK	*I'm exhausted*	
NEW TALK	night night, time for some body rejuvenation	
e.g. OLD TALK	*I'm fat!*	
NEW TALK	I'm getting leaner and keener!	

Go on, have some fun!!

Step 3 (Make Time)

If I had a dollar for every time a client said, 'I don't have time,' I'd be rolling in it. Make time; your future health depends on it. It's not that I don't believe that you think you don't have time but you have the same 24 hours that we all have. Some of you have kids and a job and a house to clean and after-school clubs and bills to pay and food to buy and cook and the plumber to call. I get it: you are busy. Trust me here – if you didn't have kids you wouldn't miraculously have more time. You'd fill that too. Here are a few ways to find some extra time:

Get Out Of Bed!

Do you really need nine hours' sleep? Not all of you sleep nine hours, but I know that some of you who 'don't have time' do. There is no rule. Professor Jim Horne, director of Loughborough University's Sleep Research Centre says that we don't all need eight hours' sleep each night. "It's nonsense. It's like saying everybody should have size eight shoes, or be five foot eight inches." Apparently, what really matters is whether we feel fresh and alert during the day. Prime Minister Margaret Thatcher was known for needing only five hours a night and ran the country. Professor Horne believes the amount of sleep we require is likely down to our genes and what we are accustomed to.

So if you slept for six hours, went off to work and performed well without feeling the pain of dragging yourself from hour to hour, then six hours is good for you. Have you ever noticed that what you have to do each morning directly impacts how tired you are, regardless of how much sleep you've had? It's 9.00 a.m. and today you have an office meeting that is sure to bore you to tears. You've had six hours sleep, you've pressed the snooze button three times and it's yawn, yawn and yawn throughout the day. Now *flip it...* It's 9.00 a.m. and you're meeting friends at this fabulous new breakfast spot in town to discuss an exciting new idea for a shared business, over a plateful of yummy pancakes with gorgeous organic maple syrup (good Canadian that I am). You've had just six hours sleep. Woohoo... Is that you I hear singing in the shower? Food for thought.

Too Much Sleep

The studies really seem to suggest that we need between five and ten hours (*hypersomnia*) but within those limits it's really anything goes, as long as you feel refreshed during the day. 'If people get less than five hours, or more than ten hours of sleep, it increases their mortality.' (Michael Breus, author of *Beauty Sleep*)

There is some interesting research on hypersomnia. My own experience concurs. When I get more than eight hours sleep, I feel sluggish. When I make myself rise between

6.00-6.30 a.m., although a little *painful*, I always feel super-charged those days. Besides, if I sleep too much I hear my father's words ringing in my ears: "You're sleeping your life away!" That thought is enough to get even the laziest out of bed.

Healthy Night-time Rituals

I spent some time when I was growing up with great family friends Barbara and John from Newfoundland. They were fond of tucking us in and whispering, "See you in the…" and we'd all chime, "morning." It was lovely. My family still say it today. Night-time rituals are good. That's why we use them with kids. Little snack, bath, hairbrush, story and then bed – same time each night. Or perhaps this is more familiar: microwave meal, bottle of red, idiot box, feeling tired, exhaustion and flop.

Consider a ritualised bath or shower an hour before bed. I always had a bath before bed when I was younger and I still find that I love a bath, along with some nice fragrant oils and the lights turned low. To get a good night's sleep you may need to consider cutting out the stimulants (alcohol, caffeine, sugar) a few hours before bed. I know, you love your tea and coffee but do you love it more than a good night's sleep? You decide. A cool bedroom is also important, so turn off the radiator or turn down the heating at least an hour before bed.

You may also want to consider shutting down your brain activity a couple of hours before bedtime. That means no computer, no TV and no *How To Live The Life Of Your Dreams* books (my version of TV) before bed. Get that idiot box out of the bedroom – it's a bedroom not a cinema!

Even insomniacs can reset their natural rhythms by setting a strict getting-up time that is quite early (6.00-7.00 a.m.) and going to bed when they are truly tired and not a minute before – even if that means the first few nights are 1.00 a.m.-6.00 a.m. Insomniacs should avoid using the bedroom for anything but sleep. *No* to reading in bed and certainly *no* to the idiot box before bed. Nada! This usually gets the non-sleeper on track within just a couple of weeks. After you have re-established a healthy sleep cycle, you can join the sleepers in creating your own bedtime routine.

Step 4 (Add Three Years To Your Life)

Do you know that by the time you are 36 most of you will have lost at least three years of your life watching TV! Yikes. I actually sat down one day and computed it. On average, a person watches two hours of TV a day (likely a very conservative estimate). Here's what happens when I think too much:

2 hours TV/day x 7 days/week x 52 weeks/year (2x7x52=728)

728 hours/year ÷ 24 hours/day = 30 days

1 month lost every year!

So by the time you are 36 years of age you've lost 36 months or three years of your life. Let's say you are lucky enough to live for 84 years; that is a whopping 84 months lost or seven years of your life spent watching TV! How many of us faced with *our end* might like an extra seven years to play with? I certainly would. That little calculation had me get rid of my TV and I've been without since 2005. I highly recommend it for the inspired learners among you.

Step 5 (Practise Saying No)

'I just can't say no.' Is this you? You are the ones who come to see me in practice with chronic problems – often chronic pain. My belief is that those of you who *can't say no* have suppressed *no's* that need to get out. I'm fond of saying, "Better out than in." I believe that *yes* people are susceptible to developing chronic health issues because they never stop. Rose is a *yes* person.

Meet Rose

Rose came to see me for her long-standing posture concerns and, in particular, the fear of her developing *neck hump*. She had always known something was wrong, but never really believed

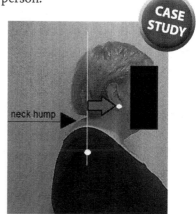

Rose

anyone could help her. Her x-rays revealed severe forward head posture with arthritis (quite advanced due to her posture). Although Rose began receiving treatment later in life than she wished she had and too late to reverse her forward head posture, her pain and stiffness have decreased dramatically. She now receives regular check-ups to help her posture from getting any worse. It is unlikely her neck hump can be corrected at this stage.

Most recently, Rose had a relapse while on holiday. When she came in to see me she said, "I don't know what's happened, I haven't done anything." She thought perhaps it was the travel but when I began to enquire, she recounted the lead-up to her trip. She was really feeling stressed out before her travels and knew that she needed to get ready for her trip and her own imminent wedding but she had offered to help a friend who was recovering from an operation. Collectively, these three things had caused her to become very stressed. Rose finds it difficult to say *no* to requests for help. She explains, "I want to help but physically I do not have the stamina."

Rose is what I affectionately call a *yes* person (aka *The Helper*). She has a hard time saying *no* to people. Do you recognise yourself in Rose? I explained to Rose that if she made herself ill from all this running about, she would be unable to help her friends or family. I suggested that we occasionally need to put ourselves first and learn to say *no*. That may be uncomfortable for many of you. Saying *no* does not make you a selfish person, it simply means that you value your health and well-being and recognise that you can't please everyone all of the time.

If you are a *Helper* like Rose, who finds it difficult to say *no*, you may find that by practising saying *no* you discover more time for taking care of yourself and, as a result, have fewer chronic health problems. I advised Rose to try telling her friend something like this: "My chiropractor Paula said I need to slow down. I get all worked up helping everyone else and sometimes forget to take care of myself. I really want to help you because I care about you. Would you understand if I saw you just once a week, as I don't want to have any further health issues? I'm practising taking care of myself – I'm not used to doing that."

The Helper – Good

You are empathetic and compassionate, encouraging, appreciative and thoughtful. You are likely very generous and helpful. You are unselfish, sincere, loving and joyful.

Helpers Beware!

You need to be needed and want others to depend on you. You often wear yourself ragged. Some *helpers* may indirectly dominate others using guilt. The suppression of your passive aggression may result in health problems. Start today. Practise saying *no*!

Step 6 (Get Moving!)

It's 7.00 a.m. – it's down to the kitchen you go for an injection of caffeine and then it's into the shower and straight out the door. You've barely had a moment's thought about your body and what it may need. What body? You mean that stiff thing I just dragged out of bed? Then it's a commute to the office and more caffeine. It's now 10.30 a.m. and your body is speaking. What it says isn't pretty – *exhausted, hate the job, hate the boss.* Now it's over to the coffee house for a croissant and latte, then emails – type – Facebook – type – Twitter – type - B-R-E-A-T-H-E. Now your body is shouting – *feed me*! Sandwich time, another latte and then a first glass of water for your stiff body – you just remembered your chiropractor said you must drink more water. Does this sound like you? Have you become an office *slouch potato*? If you are like the majority of 30-40 somethings, this is you. What ever state of slouch potato you are in, I want to help you.

Motion Is Lotion

I'm fond of saying "Motion is lotion." What I mean is that movement is lotion to your joints, just as oil is lubricant to your car engine. Children innately know what is good for them, which is why they constantly fidget. Do you ever say to yourself, "Oh to have that kind of energy," while watching children playing? Children don't walk along the street; they skip, hop, spin, run, wiggle and giggle. We could learn a lot from *our* children.

After age ten, your spinal discs (the shock absorbers between the vertebrae) become avascular (no blood supply). The discs rely on nutrients being squeezed in and out from blood vessels in the periphery (mostly the *end plate*). Body movement, or even just changing your posture, affects your disc nutrition. 'It seems feasible that alternating periods of activity and rest, and frequent posture changes, would boost the fluid exchange in the discs, hence improving their nutrition.' This may be powerful prevention for the degenerative disc disease that inevitably accompanies the typical sedentary lifestyle, often leading to low back pain, slipped discs * and stiffness.

Slipped discs don't actually slip. The gel-like material (nucleus) leaks out through cracking in the cartilage rings (annulus).

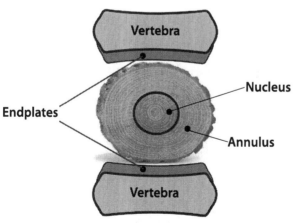

no body movement ▶ no disc nutrition ▶ disc degeneration

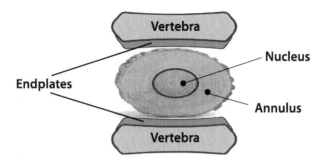

movement ▶ nutrition squeezed into disc ▶ healthy discs

Think of your spinal discs like the rings of a tree stump, with a gel-like centre (the nucleus), cartilage rings (annulus) and a cartilage end-plate or disc-like *cap*. Your body movements squeeze nutrients from the end plate, to and from your discs much like a sponge.

Sitting, The New Smoking

Dr James Levine is a researcher at the Mayo Clinic in Rochester, Minnesota and has a passion for studying how much people move. In a 1999 study he asked why some sedentary people gain more weight than other sedentary people when they eat the same amount of food. With the help of his motion-tracking underwear, he discovered that the sedentary people who didn't gain weight were the ones who unconsciously moved around more. Dr Levine's studies showed that those who gained weight sat an extra two hours a day compared to those who didn't gain weight. Those who didn't gain the weight found simple ways to move throughout the day – taking the stairs, trips to the water cooler, fidgeting at their desk and busying themselves with household chores.

We have been told, however, that those with sedentary lifestyles and jobs can offset the harm of inactivity by simply eating well and hitting the gym a few times a week for some aerobic activity. Unfortunately, new research is questioning this level of reasoning and one could compare this advice with the foolish logic that jogging could offset the risk of a pack-a-day smoking habit. In this respect, sitting is the new smoking.

Marc Hamilton is an *inactivity researcher* and warns that the inactivity of sitting has our muscles go dead. Our calorie burning plunges and our insulin effectiveness drops 40% in just 24 hours, increasing our risk of Type 2 diabetes. Alpa Patel, an epidemiologist, carried out a 14-year study on 123,000 Americans. The women in the study who spent at least six hours a day sitting had a death rate 40% higher (20% higher for men) than those who sat for three hours or less. The conclusion seems to be that being sedentary and sitting all day at the office is bad for your health even if you hit the gym.

The good news is that you can counteract the risks of sitting all day at the office with constant small movements throughout the day – fidget, stir and wiggle. Roll your shoulders, turn your neck, wiggle your legs, turn your ankles and get up and walk every hour. This is what I call *active sitting*. You need to make exercise easy. If the thought of heading to the gym fills you with horrified visions of Lycra and uber fit 20-somethings with sweaty perfect bodies, then the gym may not be the place for you. You don't need a gym membership to get healthy.

HEALTHY TIP

Here are some of my top tips for free easy exercise:

- *Park farther away (save on gas and save the planet at the same time)*

- *Walk up and down escalators (quite a workout if using the London Underground)*

- *When staying in hotels, walk at least four floors to and from your room*

- *Always walk with purpose (at a good pace)*

- *Use a backpack so you can swing your arms and get the most benefit from walking*

- *Vacuum like you mean it (using a fencing position and use your legs, not your back)*

- *Walk, don't drive to the corner store (yes, even when it's raining)*

- *Take small steps two at a time*

- *Fidget (wiggle in your chair, on the train and on a plane)*

The **1-Minute Workout**

Dr Levine tells us that the one-hour daily gym session does not make up for the dangers of sitting all day in the office. For those of you three-times-a-week gym goers who consider yourselves healthy, this may come as a shock. It appears that your compressed office bodies need a chance to recover after each hour of sitting. It is for that reason I created the 1-Minute Workout (see **Resources**). I think most of you could easily commit to 60 seconds, eight times a day at work. Is it even possible that eight minutes stretched out over the course of a day's work has more benefit than 60 minutes at the gym? Well, Professor Jamie Timmons believes so.

In a BBC 2 television programme *The Truth About Exercise*, Jamie Timmons explains that high-intensity interval training (HIT) is a possible alternative to traditional cardiovascular exercise and just three minutes of HIT a week for four weeks could provide significant change to our health. The HIT research was carried out on BBC presenter Michael Mosley. The research suggests that we may benefit more from 60-second exercise bursts (which are highly fatiguing) than lengthy workout sessions due to the amount of muscle tissue used in HIT (up to four times more than with ordinary moderate aerobic exercise). This is good news for the chronic *slouch potato*.

Now I'm definitely not advocating this approach to exercise exclusively. I feel this type of exercise research is just too new (and too darn convenient), but taking a 60-second exercise break each hour is a very good start for many of you. Of course all those hours spent sitting play havoc with your posture – round shoulders, forward head and the dreaded *neck hump.*

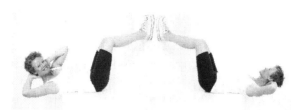

CHAPTER ELEVEN

You're Looking Fabulous!

So you're ready to look fabulous, hurray! You've already learned so much – made a commitment (you bought the book) and created a *new possibility* for your health and posture. You understand *normal* posture and have a good idea of your own *posture type*. You have seen how it is that you got to be this way and understand that it has little to do with your genes or age and a lot to do with your lifestyle.

You are going to need support and you will most likely desire a *vitalistic* full-body approach. You are ready to make time because you know that waiting is a sure path to relationship breakdown, chronic health problems, plummeting confidence and premature ageing. You can begin to trust your body and manage your own pain threshold without drugs. You have a better idea of your *real age* and how you can begin to grow young. So all that is missing is a plan for your *game*; all successful plans have three fundamental *rules*.

Make A Plan

'There is no writer's block,
just bad planning.'

Mindy Gibbins-Klein
The Book Midwife

I've never bought a lottery ticket for myself. I grew up picking numbers out of an envelope for my father who had hopes of winning big but that is the closest I ever came to buying a ticket for myself. I simply don't want to win the lottery. Yes, you read that right. Money to me is just a prize that tells me I'm winning a game. If I get money because I am winning the game, then everything I spend my money on I enjoy. If money was simply handed to me, then my game would be over. Boring! Planning is crucial in the *game* of success, but before you make a plan for your game you have to know what game you are playing.

Is your game to get a sexy flexible body, have energy to play with your kids, start a new hobby or take a dream holiday? Or is your game to see just how much health and vitality you can squeeze out of your body in this lifetime? That's my game! Whatever your game, all games have rules – a *plan* if you like. There is a starting point (fatigue, stress, aches, pains, low self-esteem) and there is a finish to the game (I'll let you define that). In order to go from start to finish, you need a plan.

'If we set off on a road trip without any identified destination, the trip itself is unlikely to be much fun.

If we do not know where we are going or even where we want to go, every fork in the road becomes a site of ambivalence – neither turning left nor turning right seems a good choice as we do not know whether we want to end up where these roads lead. So instead of focusing on the landscape, the scenery, the flowers on the side of the road, we are consumed by hesitation and uncertainty. If we have a destination in mind… we are free to focus our full attention on making the most of where we are.' (Tal Ben-Shahar author of *Happier)*

Top Three Planning Rules

Planning works. Poor planning or no planning does not work. If I didn't have a plan for this book it wouldn't have been written. When it comes to planning, there are three fundamental elements to your planning success. Your plan must be **simple**, **convenient** and **fun.** You can add a fourth and that is to make your plan *time-bound.*

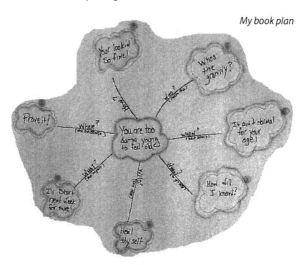

My book plan

Keep It Simple

When I work with my clients we start slow, ridiculously so. I want you to succeed so start simple and build on that. I exercise every day but that isn't what I want for you just yet. Start out with a simple list of all the things you are already doing well and not so well – that is the **Now** column. Then make a list of things to include in your **Want To Be** column. Consider where you want to be in one week, one month and one year from now. Be specific (*feeling sexy in my swimsuit* vs. *slim*; *waking at 6.45 a.m.* vs *more energy*). Create a list of all the things you need to work into the plan to attain your goals and get to where you **want to be**. Put this list into some kind of chronological order that makes sense to you. **Your plan** may include:

- *Drink water (be specific: three, five, eight glasses?)*
- *Drink only one coffee a day*
- *Bed at 10.30 p.m., wake at 6.30 a.m. (that is eight hours by the way!)*
- *Book a Skype Consultation (see Resources)*
- *Make a pot of healthy stew each Sunday*
- *Join a salsa class and go to first class next Friday*
- *Learn how to diaphragm breathe (video on posturevideos.com)*
- *Write down my WHY and stick it on bathroom mirror*
- *Begin the Posturecise DVD by _____ (see Resources)*
- *Have a 20-minute power walk Monday and Friday*

NOW ▶	YOUR PLAN ▶	WANT TO BE
1.		
2.		
3.		
4.		
5.		
6.		
7.		

Get absolutely everything you can think of down on paper. Your **Now** column may already include things like drinking water, eight hours sleep, five fruit and veg, exercise, happy marriage, good social life. Your **Want To Be** column may list losing ten pounds, wearing a bikini, going swimming with your kids, stopping pain medication, getting up at 7.00 a.m., regularly watching my posture videos, reducing your neck hump, booking a spa detox weekend, feeling flexible on waking – the more specific the better. Now obviously you aren't going to launch straight in and tackle the entire list. You may have tried this approach in the past, only to find you gave up. It felt too much like hard work. Keep it simple and start slowly. Build the timescale into your plan: Week 1 (drink five glasses of water daily, take posture quiz, 20-minute *purposeful* walk). Week 2 (Week 1 + Skype Consultation + salsa class). Week 3 (Week 1 + Week 2 + begin Posturecise DVD). Your plan should span a minimum of 12 weeks. I believe this is a reasonable time frame to establish new lifelong habits.

Some of you will feel motivated enough to go it alone but for those of you who choose to ask for support, remember to choose a vitalistic whole body *structural* approach. I think my posture services are excellent. They are designed from hundreds of case studies that span more than a decade. Because I understand the structure and physics of the spine, I can often help you get results that last. I learned to correct my own stubborn posture (even with an *untreatable* condition of the spine) so I know that it works!

Make It Convenient

We all have 24 hours in a day but still we love to complain that we don't have time – but we all have the same 24 hours! Some of you have children, you own a business, volunteer your time or care for sick family. I get it: you are busy. If you want results you had better make your planning convenient.

Body movement (exercise) needs to be a daily practice and not just a rushed three visits a week in a packed gym either. Make your body movement practise frequent, daily and convenient – mornings if you possibly can. Morning may not be the best time to exercise in terms of your body's state of readiness but if you rely on evening exercise it becomes very easy to let it slip because you are tired. If you choose to exercise in the mornings, you need to warm your body up first with a shower or some easy marching on the spot. As I write this book, I am in the planning stages of releasing my own morning posture routines on DVD (see **Resources**).

Find ways to exercise during the day. Park farther away, take the stairs, walk the escalator, fidget in your office chair and do my 1-Minute Workout every hour at work. Do chin tucks while you wait in the post office. Roll your ankles when you sit down. Do some pelvic circles when you stand up. I'm serious – keep wiggling all day long and check out our posture videos for more ideas for *easy exercise.* Have you ever noticed that kids never stop moving? They are flexible, strong and playful and typically sleep the sleep of angels – hmm.

Avoid distractions at all costs. Put this into your plan. I've got a great distraction habit: I de-clutter and organise. This is a sneaky one because everybody knows you need to be clutter-free to clear your mind and free up your energy. Watch out for this one. Other common distractions: your mobile phone, eating, paying bills, sorting paper and email. Decide on specific times each day to check email and don't check email before bed as you can't address emergencies at that time and it is a recipe for insomnia. Try a 'no computer before bed' rule to slow your brain down. Make a list of your Top Three Distractions and work them into your plan. Make some rules and stick to them!

Make It Fun

This is the best part. Make your plan fun. If you literally drag yourself to the gym and then desperately watch the timer on the bike or treadmill, then my guess is you're not having much fun. Even if you haven't exercised your entire life and find it hurts every time you try, remember this: exercise stimulates the production of chemicals known as endorphins (your natural antidepressants). The natural *highs* you get from regular exercise will more than offset any discomfort you initially have to endure.

Just about anything counts as exercise. Turn on the music and dance around cleaning your house if that turns you on. I need variety. I begin each morning with a 30-minute posture routine. It's my routine that gets this 40-something body ready for the day ahead. I exercise on a blue padded mat below a large skylight and marvel at the sky. This works for me – it's my special time of day.

I usually take one five-mile walk into town each week – arms swinging, pulse dancing. I often use these walks to practise speaking things out loud that I'm working on. In the summer I play softball twice a week. I hadn't played softball since I was a child and last year I joined a local team and absolutely love it. My body ached when I began but I knew I'd build up to the point where I didn't feel like a granny every time I played. I also ride my adult-sized scooter four miles once a week to see my chiropractor for an *adjustment.* I incorporate exercise into my life – I make it **simple, convenient** and **fun**!

> *Take lessons in something you always wanted to learn (fencing, tennis, archery, skiing, swimming, squash, golf, dancing, roller blading). Join a dance class (Zumba, Street Dance, Belly Dancing, Pole Dancing, Salsa). Buy a new toy (scooter, hacky sack, balance board, adult trike, skateboard, football, basketball). Do something out of character and have some fun. Fun will get it done!*

HEALTHY TIP

Detox Your Life

I am guessing that you might like to shave a few years off, but you'd like to keep drinking wine with dinner most evenings, having your daily latte and muffin, lunchtime chocolate bar and hours of idle TV viewing. Guess what? You can have all of this and still be healthy! Oh no, sorry, did I get your hopes up? It isn't possible. According to Albert Einstein, the very definition of insanity is 'Doing the same thing over and over again and expecting different results.' Amen to that!

The spiritual teacher, Osho, describes *pleasure seeking* as our most animal of instincts and the least likely to provide happiness, joy and bliss. You may find immediate pleasure in the glass of wine, the hour of television or the piece of cake or the wad of cash, but when they are gone so is the fleeting happiness. He says that pleasure is always outside of us (external) and requires some *thing* to provide the happiness. True happiness, joy and bliss he explains is found within, when we are being true to our real nature. If you are like many, have lost that sense of who you are, look to your childhood and the things that brought you joy. Osho suggests that it is there that you will find your bliss.

So your journey to health and well-being is likely to be successful and lifelong if you find the inner joy connected with your health. When I am exercising, I am almost in a state of meditation. The time seems to melt away and I am blissed-out. Not always, because sometimes life takes over and I remember all the things I need to do and I lose my bliss, but for the most part I love moving my body and connecting with *me*.

Emotional Detox

In order to enjoy regaining your health you may need a whole *new view of health*. 'We all want to be healthy and happy. We desire more vitality, more energy, more attractiveness and as we get older we spend more time thinking about our health. Often when we think of health we think of how we would like to change our current state of health – from smoking to not smoking, from being large to being thin, from not exercising to exercising, or from eating junk food to eating "healthy" food. Before we consider becoming healthier, I suggest that we first need a new view of health, a paradigm shift, a *new possibility* for our health and ourselves.' (From *Abundant Health*)

A *new view of health* begins with your current view and grows from there. Recall Ellen Langer's study on hotel maids. She found that when she explained to the maids that the exercise they were getting from their work counted as real exercise, their health improved. The only thing that changed was their mindset (how *mindful* they were of their own state of health).

There has been ongoing research into the health benefits of *mindfulness* using meditation since the early 1970s. The majority of the research has focused on the potential benefits to cardiovascular health. A study conducted by researchers at the Department of Internal Medicine at the University of Kentucky established that the regular practice of meditation may have the potential to reduce blood pressure by 4.7 mm Hg, which can subsequently reduce the risk of high blood pressure, heart attack and stroke. Other areas of meditation research that show promising results have been mental health (ADHD and anxiety), memory, addictions, brain function, pain control and asthma.

Meditation may have the potential to reduce blood pressure

Your view of health (what you think and believe) is powerful. Do you say: '*Nothing ever works for me, I tried but I can't, I don't have time, I hate exercise* or *it's just too much like hard work*'? I have heard it all from my clients. Daniel Priestley, author of *Become A Key Person Of Influence,* frequently says, "You get what you pitch for." In other words, if your *pitch* about life is *I don't have time...* guess what? You get what you pitch for... **no time**! Changing your mindset takes practice and there are many different approaches you can try. Find one that works for you and stick with it.

Breathing

Deepak Chopra, American physician and author, is an advocate of meditation. He recommends two sessions of 20 minutes each day. Now if meditation is something you have always wanted to take on then go for it. Remember my admonishment – keep it **simple** and **convenient** and add it to your plan. I recommend starting with two weeks of one daily ten-minute session and then build on that. Don't make this too complicated (forget the candles, primordial sounds and expensive cushions). Just sit and breathe and sit some more and breathe some more. Seriously though, there is no right or wrong way to meditate.

I have found the easiest way to begin with meditation is to make it all about the breathing. Breathe in and *watch* your breath in. Breathe out and *watch* your breath out. If you are like me, you may find you are thinking about tonight's dinner or that your foot has gone to sleep. It doesn't matter. Just go back to breathe in and *watch*, breathe out and *watch*. I have never been that successful in the practice of meditation but for me my body work is my state of meditation. You may meditate painting, running, cooking, sewing or using just about anything that has the time slip away unnoticed.

Make it all about
the breathing

Visualisation

If you are a dreamer like me, it isn't hard to see your future in all its colourful, fulfilling glory. When I was renovating my chiropractic clinic and the flat above, I slept on a pull-out bed with my memory foam mattress overhanging the frame and only the dusty shell of walls remaining of what was once my home. My friends thought I was mad but I could actually visualise the entire finished flat: the whitewash floors, the mezzanine from which I am now writing, the huge skylight under which I do my daily exercise and the pine floating staircase that I designed from a picture in a magazine.

You will know if this type of mindful practice is for you. Play with it and see if it works for you. Professional athletes use visualisation and there have been studies where athletes were able to increase their muscle tone through visualisation alone. Don't count on that being your only form of exercise though – nice try!

You can use visualisation during meditation or just create the visuals around you. Make a dream board – a collage of all the things that will help you visualise your new state of health and vitality. On it you may include pictures of the body you want, the beautiful food you will cook, the country walks you will take and the dog who will join you. You could also put some inspiring words and images around your house, in your car, on your fridge or bathroom mirror. I have words and pictures drawn all over my bathroom tiles – use a non-permanent marker and have some **fun** with this!

Affirmations

What do you tell yourself regularly? What words (positive or negative) do you repeatedly use? These are affirmations. If I'm not careful, when I am really annoyed with myself, I grunt, "Paula you idiot." Not very inspiring is it? I rarely do this now but I had to really get strict with myself and see that this did nothing for my emotional health. What do you frequently say to yourself? *I'm fat*? *I'm sorry*? *I'm exhausted*? *Dummy*? *Idiot*? *Stupid*? These aren't very empowering words. If you aren't sure of the words you repeatedly use, ask someone close to you to point them out. For those words you mumble when nobody is looking, you will have to police yourself. You can choose new words to add to your daily vocabulary: *I will* vs. *I'll try; I'm sexy* vs. *I'm fat; silly goose* vs. *idiot*. Go on – remember the third rule of planning is to have **fun**!

Affirmations can also be used as a sort of mantra. Choose words that resonate for you. The kind of affirmations that don't work are ones that are so unbelievable that you almost chuckle saying them. So if *I'm healing myself, the planet and the universe* doesn't quite cut it, try to simplify. The idea of repeating an affirmation is that your brain doesn't know the difference between saying the words and the actual words. If you repeat them often enough – 50 times daily – your brain may begin to perceive those words as reality. I give you permission to play.

Try these out or write your own:

- *I'm sexy!*
- *I'm full of energy!*
- *I feel alive and well!*
- *I love moving my body!*
- *Motion is lotion (this is one of mine – lotion to your joints)*
- *I look and feel 20 years younger (humour me!)*

Chemical Detox – You Are What You Eat

'Garbage in, garbage out' – another of my mantras. If you put junk in, you can't expect your body to give you vitality and youthful energy. Your body is literally made of the food and liquid that you put in it.

It is true that all food (even the poorest quality food) will be broken down and used by your body but it is the difference between using high octane fuel and regular fuel for your car. The better the fuel, the better the performance. I could write an entire book just on food but for this book all I want you to understand is why *real food* is *best food*. Poor food quality means more sugar, sodium, additives (chemicals), hydrogenated fats (trans fats) and artificial colours.

Poor food quality affects your ideal body chemistry and the workings of your finely tuned systems. Processed and ready-made packaged meals contain few, if any, nutritional ingredients. They are bulked out with cornflour, processed potato, egg and milk products, hydrogenated oils, saturated fats and sugars and then made to taste better with the addition of herbs and spices, high salt, monosodium glutamate (MSG) and more sugar. They contain artificial colours (to make it look more appealing), preservatives (for long shelf life) and artificial flavourings (more chemicals).

When your diet lacks fresh fruit and vegetables, your intake of essential nutrients is close to zero. Your intake of dietary fibre is also low to non-existent and that places you at risk of strokes from high blood pressure, Type 2 diabetes (from irregular blood sugar levels), heart attacks (from raised cholesterol levels) and colon cancer as you are unable to process the waste products without sufficient dietary fibre. You will experience more frequent illness as your immune system is compromised and you'll have a greater chance of developing other forms of cancer as your levels of antioxidants (found in fresh fruit and vegetable) are low.

You are more likely to experience premature ageing with early onset arthritis and other inflammatory diseases as your overall body acidity rate increases (recall the importance of an alkaline blood pH). Processed food also leads to weight gain and obesity, further increasing the likelihood of arthritis, stroke and heart attack.

Other Chemical Stress

I want to add in two other important means of chemical stress on your body: the medications you take and the products you put on to your skin and hair. In Chapter Eight we talked about the reality of *painkilling* medication. Let's not pretend – all medication is associated with some risk. There is no safe form of medical intervention. The safest form of intervention is no intervention.

I can hear the critics screaming. I'm not saying stop taking your medication. You mustn't do that. But, you **must** be informed about what it is you are taking. Ask questions, get interested, do your own research (has this problem ever been solved without medication?) and learn to make friends with your pain. Remember that your pain serves a purpose. Your pain is your body's way of communicating that something needs to change. Do you really want to shut your body up?

Your Skin

You may already realise that your skin is an organ – the largest organ you have. Your skin acts as your immune defence from the outside world. It insulates and regulates your body temperature through sweat glands and it makes vitamin D from the sun (vital for healthy strong bones). With such an important role, you must be mindful of what you put on to your skin (make-up included). Over the last

18 months I have begun making my own skin products. This isn't as labour intensive as it sounds. I have a very thick, curly head of hair and I have always used product on my hair in an attempt to define and tame the curls. Hair gels and creams are hard to find in organic form and the few that exist have done very strange things to my curls. Definitely not attractive!

Over the last several years my scalp has become very itchy and scaly with dry skin. I was starting to notice large amounts of snow left behind on my pillow and no amount of scalp massage or hydration seemed to help. I saw a BBC television series called *Grow Your Own Drugs* by James Wong (an ethnobotanist). Wong makes natural remedies sourced from plants and I tried his remedy for my dry flaky scalp. I've now been using his hair oil (which smells divine) for about a year. All scaling has gone – no more snow. As a side effect, I've saved a fortune as I no longer purchase expensive salon gels and creams; my hair for the first time ever is soft. As an added bonus, both my hairdresser and I have noticed that I have much less grey hair. Wow! My point is that natural products have got to be better than smearing your largest organ with an expensive bottle filled with three real ingredients and a dozen extra fragrant and preserving chemicals.

If your body is in need of a chemical detox, you will know it. Your liver is the organ of detoxification and when it can no longer cope with the toxins in your body you become *intoxicated* (think hangover). If you regularly experience headaches, acne, dry itchy skin, stiff achy joints, allergies, poor digestion, anxiety, mood swings and fatigue, your body may need a detox. There are many good detox products on the market.

Move It Or Lose It!

'Everyone has a normal range of body motion. It diminishes as a consequence of inactivity. Activity restores it. Joints maintain their nutrition and their youth essentially by virtue of movement. Diminished movement ages the body prematurely,' Dr Rene Cailliet, author of *Growing Young.* Neglect your body (and its tissues), and the tissues shrivel and dry, leaving you stiff and feeling older than your years.

Your body tissues are like a sponge and like a sponge they can be kept supple or hard. Your tissues get hydrated and fed nutrients through the compression and relaxation of body movement. When your tissue isn't moved regularly, it dries out like the sponge that isn't used. Once your tissues become totally dehydrated, the fibres become sticky and fix together and this is irreversible. **Move it or lose it**. If you don't move your body and feed your tissues, eventually you will be unable to regain that flexibility and youthful ability you once had.

Stretching every day will help you maintain your flexibility and **reverse the effects of ageing**. A rubber band that is left unstretched dries up and shortens. When you then try to stretch it, it breaks. Don't let this happen to you. Fitness must be a daily process and one that you can learn to love again.

Skip The Jogging

Daily fitness is necessary to keep your body pain free and full of youthful energy. You will recall that morning stiffness is a sign of *sarcopenia* – the inevitability of flesh loss that begins from roughly age 25. I am a fan of a daily morning routine appropriate for us over-30s. Some stretching, strengthening, posture and breathing with a healthy mix of activity during the week. I am not a big fan of jogging over the age of 35.

As it turns out, once you've passed age 35 there are downsides to jogging that begin to mount up. One conclusion authorities such as Dr Cailliet have reached regarding jogging is that it is best before 35. Our tendons and ligaments are more resilient before this age, which means less strain bearing down on our cartilage during running. He cautions that it is not in your best interest to work out as hard as you can (after age 35), no matter how good you might feel at the time. *Jogging* is carried out in a more upright position than *running* (which is preferable to jogging), the back more arched and more weight being passed down through the hips, knees and feet.

The good news is that rapid walking burns more calories than jogging the same distance and works the upper body as well, all without the damaging effects of the repeated impact to which jogging subjects us. If you are absolutely insistent on jogging, make sure you don't fall into one of these categories:

- *Bunions*
- *Fallen arches*
- *Knock knees or bowed legs*
- *A short leg*
- *Scoliosis (curvature of the spine)*
- *Flat feet*
- *Overweight (although I know this would be a tempting way to lose it)*
- *History of slipped disc*
- *Hypermobile joints (very bendy)*

There are plenty of jogging alternatives. Walking, or purposeful walking as I like to call it, is my favourite. I'm about the fastest walker I know. Swimming is fantastic, biking great, or get yourself a big kid's scooter and add the element of fun. Try my posture videos –many of you write and tell me how much you enjoy them. If you prefer the support and the convenience of doing your exercise routine from home with a teacher,
I am certain you will enjoy Posturecise
– as seen on our website (see Resources).

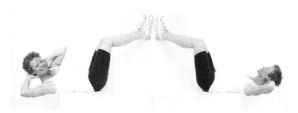

CHAPTER TWELVE

How Long Will It Take?

'How long will it take?' has to be the most common question that I receive by email. Here is my answer but I warn you, you may not like it: "It takes as long as it takes." I know, that seems quite vague and you want specifics. Do this *one magic* exercise and you will look and feel youthful forever more, but there is no quick fix! Sorry. Exercise and body movement must be a way of life and one you can learn to look forward to and enjoy – I promise you that.

Don't Give Up

You must have **realistic expectations** so that you don't give up. Some of you may start to see changes in the first few days and for others it may take several weeks. You improve your results and the speed at which you obtain them by remembering to consider your lifestyle and beginning to detox your life alongside your new exercise regime. Go back now and revise your plan if you need to.

When advising my clients on the length of time it will take to see changes (fewer aches and pains, more energy, better sleep, attractive posture, more confidence, less stress, improved flexibility and strength), I always consider these five things:

- *Your history of trauma*

- *Your current body weight*

- *Your lifestyle (physical, chemical and emotional stress)*

- *Your history of fitness*

- *Your x-ray results (amount of wear and tear... osteoarthritis)*

- **Bonus** - *Your motivation and commitment to your plan*

If you are no stranger to fitness, have good nutrition, supportive relationships, aren't overweight and have no wear in your joints, you have every reason to believe you will start seeing noticeable changes in just days! One man shared his 24-hour success story with me:

'It was a good morning. I found you. I watched some of your videos. What's so good about that? Here it is...
I have been suffering with shoulder pain for months.
I'm not a guy that runs off to the doctor at the first sign of pain. In this case, I finally went. "Here," he said, "take this prescription." I woke up this morning and

immediately went into my erect, head back posture. No pain. This is the second day. Something as simple as that, Paula. I'm telling you that I suffered for months with this shoulder pain and in a few minutes you corrected it. My doctor was going to feed me a steady diet of pain pills and muscle relaxants. I have been pain free all day because of you. You have made a believer out of me. Your presentation style makes a viewer want to watch to hear what you have to say about the topic. I thank you again and I will follow you and your videos until the day I check out.'

(Steve Mallon, author of The Path To Glory)

Fake It "til You Feel It!

There is no getting around the side effects of changing your health and ultimately how well you age. It's going to hurt, **but** it won't hurt for long. Let's face it, most of you already had aches and pains when you bought this book, so a little bit longer isn't so hard to tolerate. Remember to keep your plan **simple**, **convenient** and **fun** and stick with it by getting some support. Until you actually start seeing and feeling the results, I recommend that you simply *fake it 'til you feel it*!

Remember how Ellen Langer's hotel maids lowered their blood pressure by 10% by changing only their mindset and recall the study that showed us we could convince the brain of our future success just by adopting a more upright posture? Well, that is just great news because until you actually start to get the results that others notice (and you will), you can simply fake it and convince your mind of its success by learning some sneaky posture confidence tricks.

Posture Confidence

Your health and body posture speak volumes about you. How confident and healthy do you feel? One sign of poor health is poor posture. How you hold your body is often a reflection of how you feel about yourself. Not only do you look more attractive with upright posture but science is beginning to show us that our brains are more capable of positivity when in an upright stance.

I recently viewed a BBC documentary on television called *Virgin School* – I couldn't resist. It concerned a 26-year-old male virgin who travels to Amsterdam to become... well yes, a non-virgin. The poor man's posture was so atrocious I couldn't help but think 'no wonder'. Actually, I thought the young man was a good chap and nice looking. I just couldn't understand why nobody even considered helping him with his terrible posture. Surely this would have moved him miles in terms of his self-confidence and perhaps ultimately his luck with the ladies!

Posture and body language is almost a speciality in itself. What does your posture say about you? Or rather, what do other people think your posture says about you? What impression do they form about you? Now here is a question for you: Have you ever seen a confident person with terrible posture? Exactly! There are some basics when it comes to faking your posture confidence. Fake it first, feel it later. Here are my top ten ways to *speak* confidence through posture:

1 **No one likes a fidget**. Stop the nervous habits. Get your hands away from your mouth. Stop the feverish texting. Just be still. Confident people rarely look nervous and fidgety.

2 **Keep your legs still**. I can't help but watch all the hyperactive young men and women who sit on the London Underground, plugged into their iPods, legs vibrating at 90mph. Watch out for this one.

3 **Uncross your arms**. Crossed arms look cold, nervous, on guard and defensive. There is even a theory that this is a lazy position for your central nerve system. Don't know what to do with your arms? Try to just let them hang comfortably at your sides. Just keep practising and watch how often you do this. Uncross your legs too – your pelvic posture will improve.

4 **Don't look down**. My friends don't believe it when I tell them I am shy. I am – ask my mother. I learned a long time ago how to fake confidence with good

posture. Over time, I have become more confident. Not looking down is something I still have to practise. I play a little game with myself:

I walk down the street and someone is approaching and instead of staring down at the ground, I make gentle eye contact (don't stare, that's just weird). I make myself the last to look away. This is really hard for me. I get so uncomfortable, I just want to look away fast and sometimes I still do. Try this and you will find a whole world of people, just like you and me, who are naturally shy.

5 **Smile**! Have you ever noticed that even the funniest looking person looks attractive with a winning smile? Apparently, children smile 400 times a day compared to us adults, at a measly 15 times. When you smile it shows that you have nothing to worry about, even if you do. It warms the hearts of others and even fake smiles trigger the release of endorphins (your body's natural painkillers and antidepressants). Try smiling at yourself regularly in the bathroom mirror – go on, I dare you!

6 **Clean up**. This may be obvious but do you do it? Do you only look extra special nice when you are meeting up with friends or do you do it for yourself too? When was the last time you treated yourself to a new hairstyle, outfit, facial or colonic irrigation (haven't tried this yet but it's all the detox rage apparently). Try

dressing up a little, putting on your favourite scent just to stay in. It's amazing how good it feels to look in the mirror and find someone attractive.

7 Stand tall. Most of you will have forgotten how to stand tall due to the inevitability of our sedentary lifestyles. Try this: Think of a great big balloon attached to your chest (at the breast bone), lifting your chest. At the same time, imagine there is a string attached to your head, gently lengthening your spine as you tuck your chin inward giving you a slight double chin – sorry. Standing up straight has less to do with throwing your shoulders back and more to do with decompressing and lengthening your spine. This should feel relaxed and natural but may take a little concentration when you begin. You can find a video of me showing you *How To Gain Height Naturally* on posturevideos.com.

8 Stop the limp wrist. This is a total pet peeve of mine. The limp-wristed spaghetti handshake. If this is you, stop it! I would struggle hiring someone who shook my hand with only the tips of their *please don't bite me* fingers. Don't overcompensate and squeeze the life out of someone's hand either. Be confident but don't be strange. Make full hand to hand contact; meet thumb web to thumb web and give a firm, not powerful, squeeze. Don't linger… that's weird too. Better a cold, moist, nervous but confident handshake than a limp wrist any day.

9 Take up space. Men take up space; women are polite. Women need to stop making themselves so small (with the leg cross and wrap-around technique) and men need not spread their legs to China. Both men and women should practise taking up a little space – it shows confidence. You really don't need your legs pressed up tightly together (you can neatly tuck in a skirt) and this goes for walking too.
Don't shuffle. Stride confidently.

10 Slow down. You may have a hectic life but if you slow down and take note of your breathing you will be more efficient and not look like a nervous wreck. If you don't remember how to breathe (many of my clients start as chest breathers), place one hand over your chest and the other over your belly (while lying on your back) and spend five minutes a day breathing down into your diaphragm until your lower hand begins to rise with each breath. This takes practise over several days before the underused diaphragm muscle kicks in.

Diaphragm breathing

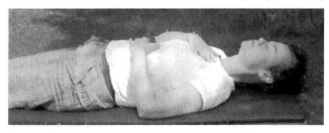

You're Ready – Piece Of Cake!

This is the end of my book and in celebration I just had a nice big piece of toffee cake at Marks and Spencer. But now all that remains is the memory and a sugary residue in my mouth. You can have this book be your piece of cake or you can have it mark the beginning of a whole new way of being. How many books on health have you read? Don't let this book be just another yummy piece of cake, soon to be forgotten.

It's time for action and this is where the **fun** and the hard work begin. I want you to succeed and I am so confident that you can, if you just start **now**. Regaining good health should be your primary objective if you want to modify the physical and cosmetic effects of ageing. When you fall off the wagon, notice and then have a little word with yourself and jump straight back on. Remind yourself of your *why*. Was it that dream back-packing holiday 12 months from now? Was it the London to Paris bike ride? Maybe it was simply to be the parent to your children that you've always dreamed you would be – the one who jumped in the pool, hopped on a bike, ran around the garden and still had energy to cook a lovely meal. Be very clear on your *why*.

You have a plan or you are at least ready to create yours. Remember your plan is to be **simple**, **convenient** and **fun**. Don't bypass fun. Get that pole dancing class in there. Buy yourself a frisbee, a hula-hoop or try a scooter if you're a bit of a tomboy like me!

Begin to detox your life and enjoy how you start to feel. Don't just focus on your physical body. Notice that you are sleeping better, thinking more clearly, smiling more often and waking without feeling old. Celebrate your *mini wins* – drinking four extra glasses of water, walking up the escalator, playing Scrabble instead of watching TV and going two whole weeks without taking any painkillers or calling yourself fat! These are big things – don't overlook them.

By now, you have a much better understanding of your health and posture and what went wrong. You understand that your thoughts can change your body and that your body can change your thoughts, even if initially you have to fake it until you feel it. You are ready to ask for help and using our posture services may be easier than going it alone. Start **now** and learn to trust your body's ability to heal itself. Make friends with your pain and always, always remember your magnificence. If all you have right now is a small belief, then start with that. You can believe yourself healthy until one day you find that you have transformed – you feel and look great and others notice. You are oozing posture confidence, standing taller and looking a good deal younger. Now that is something to celebrate!

For those of you who want ongoing support, you can join others on our website page devoted to this book. Share your stories, challenges and frustrations and celebrate your wins!

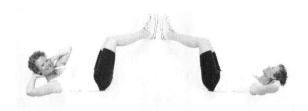

Further Resources
found at **www.posturevideos.com**

Free ebook **(Seven Biggest Mistakes People Make Correcting Posture)** join our newsletter to receive

1-Minute Workout - posturevideos.com/1-minute-workout

Coaching - www.posturedoctor.com

Posturecise (DVD) - correct your posture - home page

Posture Analysis - home page

Posture Quiz - pos-tur-o-me-ter - home page

Posture Videos - home page

Skype Consultation - home page

Social Media

Facebook - **www.facebook.com/posturedoctor**

Twitter   - **@thatpaulamoore**

YouTube - **www.youtube.com/posturevideos**

LinkedIn - **www.linkedin.com/in/posturevideos**

Comments & Questions - **ask@posturevideos.com**

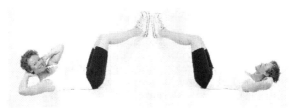

Bibliography

1. Andersen, J. W., and Liu, C., and Kryscio, R. J. (2008). 'Blood pressure response to transcendental meditation: a meta-analysis.' Am J Hypertens. 21(3), 310-6.

2. April 12, 2007. 'Why Should We Have Eight Hours Sleep?' BBC News. http://news.bbc.co.uk.

3. Bagnall, K.M., and Harris, P. F., and Jones, P. R. M. (1977). 'A radiographic study of the human fetal spine.' J Anat, 124, 791-802.

4. Ben-Shahar, T. (2008). 'Happier.' New York, New York: McGraw-Hill Professional.

5. Breus, M. (2007). 'Beauty Sleep: Look Younger, Lose Weight, and Feel Great Through Better Sleep.' Reprint edition. New York, New York: Plume Books.

6. Brinol, P., and Petty, R., and Wagner, B. (2009). 'Body posture effects on self-evaluation: A self-validation approach.' European Journal of Social Psychology. 39(6), 1053–1064.

7. Buchheld, N., and Grossman, P. and Walach, H. (2001). 'Measuring mindfulness in insight meditation (vipassana) and meditation-based psychotherapy: The development of the Freiburg Mindfulness Inventory (FMI).' Journal for Meditation and Meditation Research.1, 11-34.

8. Cailliet, R. (1989). Growing Young. London: Grafton Books.

9. Cohen, J. S. (2001). Overdose The Case Against the Drug Companies. 1st ed. New York, New York: Penguin Putnam.

10. Crum, A.J., and Landger, E. J. (2007). 'Mind-set matters: exercise and the placebo effect.' Psychol Sci. 2007 18(2), 165-71.

11. Farrant, S. (2007). Vital Truth: Accessing the possibilities of unlimited health. Springville, Utah:Vervante.

12. Ferriss, T. (2007). The 4-Hour Work Week. London: Vermilion.

13. Gagnon, J. et al. (1996). 'The Heritage Family Study: quality assurance and quality control.' Ann Epidemiol. 6(6), 520-529.

14. Glassman, S. D., and Bridwell, K., and Dimar, J. R., and Horton, W., and Berven, S., and Schwab, F. (2005). 'The Impact of Positive Sagittal balance (Forward Head Posture) in Adult Spinal Deformity.' Spine. 30(18), 2024-9.

15. Hamilton, M. T., and Hamilton, D. G., and Zderic, T. W. (2007). 'Role of Low Energy Expenditure and Sitting in Obesity, Metabolic Syndrome, Type 2 Diabetes and Cardiovascular Disease.' Diabetes. 56, 2655-2667.

16. Holford, P. (2007). 'The Holford 9-Day Liver Detox .' London: Piatkus.

17. Horizon-'The Truth About Exercise.' April 13, 2012. BBC 2: Episode 8 of 15. Television.

18. Hublin, C., Markku, P., Markku, K., Jaakko, K. (2007). 'Sleep and mortality: a population-based 22-year follow-up study.' Sleep, 30(10),1245-1253.

19. Kado, D. M., Huang, M., and Barrett-Connor, E., and Greendale, G. A. (2004). 'Hyperkyphotic Posture Predicts Mortality in Older Community-dwelling Men and Women: A Prospective Study.' J Am Geriatr Soc. 52 (10), 1662—1667.

20. Jan, 2012. 'Osteoporosis: Peak Bone Mass in Women.' NIH Osteoporosis and Related Bone Diseases - National Resource Center. http://www.niams.nih.gov/Health_Info/Bone/ osteoporosis/bone_mass.asp.

21. Lennon, J., and Sheeley, N., and Roger, K. C., and Matta, W., and Cox, R., and Simpson, W. F. (1994). 'Postural and Respiratory Modulation of Autonomic Function, Pain and Health.' Am J Pain Manag. 4, 36-39.

22. Lipton, B. (2011). The Biology of Belief: Unleashing the Power of Consciousness, Matter & Miracles. London: Hay House UK.

23. National Institute of Arthritis and Musculo-skeletal and Skin Diseases. (2011). 'Questions and Answers about Growth Plate Injuries.' http://www.niams.nih.gov.

24. Oct 5, 2009. 'Body Posture Affects Confidence In Your Own Thoughts, Study Finds.' Science Daily. www.sciencedaily.com.

25. Oliver, J., and Middleditch, A. (1991). Functional Anatomy of the Spine. Oxford: Butterworth-Heinemann.

26. O'Meara, C. et al. (2010). 'Abundant Health.' Australia: Penguin Group.

27. Patel, A. V. (2010). 'Leisure Time Spent Sitting in Relation to Total Mortality in a Prospective Cohort of US Adults.' American Journal of Epidemiology. *Correspondence to Dr. Alpa V. Patel, Epidemiology Research Program, American Cancer Society, 250 Williams Street NW, Atlanta, GA 30303.

28. Priestley, Daniel. (2010). Become a Key Person of Influence: The 5 Step Sequence to becoming one of the most highly valued and highly paid people in your industry. Hertfordshire: Ecademy Press.

29. Revill, J. April 9, 2006. 'Sleep – Our New Obsession.' The Observer. www.guardian.co.uk.

30. Riso, D. R. (1995). Discovering Your Personality Type. Revised edition. Boston, Massachusetts: Houghton Mifflin.

31. Souza, T. A. (2001). Differential Diagnosis And Management For The Chiropractor. 2nd ed. New York, New York: Aspen Publishers Inc.

32. 'Virgin School.' Channel 4. May 15, 2007. Television.

33. Vlahos, J. Apr 14, 2011. 'Is Sitting A Lethal Activity?' The New York Times Magazine. www.nytimes.com.

34. Wannamethee, S. G., and Shaper, G., and Lennon, L., and Whincup, P. H. (2006). 'Height Loss in Older Men: Associations With Total Mortality and Incidence of Cardiovascular Disease.' Arch Intern Med. 166, 2546-2552.

35. Wikipedia. May, 2012. 'History of Depression.' http://en.wikipedia.org/wiki/History_of_depression.

36. Wong, J. (2010). 'Grow Your Own Drugs.' London: Collins.

37. World Health Organization. (1946). 'Preamble to the Constitution of the World Health Organization as adopted by the International Health Conference.' Official Records of the World Health Organization, no. 2, p. 100.

38. Yochum, T.R., and Rowe, L.J. (1996). Essentials of Skeletal Radiology. 2nd ed. Vol 1. London: Lippincott Williams and Wilkins.

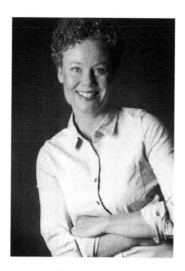

Paula Moore is a self-confessed posture addict. She is the creator of a popular video blog on posture which has received over one million youtube views. She is the author of Posture Give It To Me Straight and a co-author of Abundant Health.

A graduate of The Anglo-European College of Chiropractic, she holds a Masters and a fellowship in the field of posture science. She has appeared in The Mail on Sunday, GMTV's Breakfast Television and on the highly regarded BBC Woman's Hour.

Paula lives by the sea in the beautiful South East where she is often seen whizzing by on her Kickbike, playing softball or eating a big piece of cake in one of Brighton's quirky cafés.

www.posturevideos.com

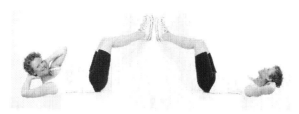

Testimonials

"It was a good morning. I found you. I watched some of your videos. What's so good about that? Here it is... I have been suffering with shoulder pain for months. I'm not a guy that runs off to the doctor at the first sign of pain. In this case, I finally went. "Here," he said, "take this prescription." I woke up this morning and immediately went into my erect, head back posture. No pain. This is the second day. Something as simple as that, Paula. I'm telling you that I suffered for months with this shoulder pain and in a few minutes you corrected it. My doctor was going to feed me a steady diet of pain pills and muscle relaxants. I have been pain free all day because of you. You have made a believer out of me. Your presentation style makes a viewer want to watch to hear what you have to say about the topic. I thank you again and I will follow you and your videos until the day I check out."

Steve Mallon, *author of The Path To Glory*

"A few months ago I noticed my posture was not all it should be. The long hours spent working at the computer were beginning to take their toll. My first reaction was 'What can I do about this?' This prompted an internet search and this is where I found Paula Moore. I have recently purchased Paula's new book, this explains the importance of good posture and details the steps you can take to correct your posture. I am at the moment following the suggested exercise routines and I do notice my posture is improving; added to this it has also given me a real awareness of my posture in day-to-day situations."

Richard Manning

"This past week I have been unable to walk with severe right thigh pain... terrible cramp-like feeling... my chiropractor thought it was sciatica... my butt cheek was so tight you could hardly touch it... then I found your video... I did the stretch and I could walk without pain... thanks so much, I had lost my job... I was so sad to think I would be like this for a long time... my life seemed to be over, could do nothing and pain pills did not touch it... it was a miracle I found your video... thanks so much."

Sandi Killian

*"Finally someone who can tell me this is a problem...
This felt so good. My regular doctor said not much
can be done for my neck lump and the severe pain I
have in my back. I have been practising doing the neck
exercises daily. I really see an improvement in pain
and the lump. Again, I thank you for helping people
with information on an issue that does not seem to be
widely discussed." Sincerely,*

Jane Seitz

*The pain has been almost debilitating. After just a few
days of following your exercises, I can move and walk
without grimacing.*

Stephen Bloch

*"I am so grateful for 'stumbling' upon Paula's videos
when I did a youtube search about forward head
posture. I have been dealing with this for years, but
only recently realised I had it. I was fortunate enough
to be able to have a conversation via Skype with
Paula to talk about my condition. She was soooo
helpful and informative. She thoroughly answered
all of my questions (what type of exercises are best,
what should I look for in a chiropractor, how long will
this correction take? etc.) and she gave me a suggested
plan of action... I only wish she was local so I could
have her as my chiropractor. But her DVDs and Skype
calls are the next best thing. Thanks, Paula!"*

Mara Grigsby

Made in the USA
Lexington, KY
02 January 2017